£17.99 *Withdrawn* *13/2/09*

Nursing the Dying Patient

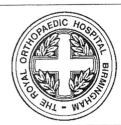

Nursing the Dying Patient

Caring in Different Contexts

John Costello

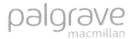

© John Costello 2004

All rights reserved. No reproduction, copy or transmission of this publication may be made without written permission.

No paragraph of this publication may be reproduced, copied or transmitted save with written permission or in accordance with the provisions of the Copyright, Designs and Patents Act 1988, or under the terms of any licence permitting limited copying issued by the Copyright Licensing Agency, 90 Tottenham Court Road, London W1T 4LP.

Any person who does any unauthorised act in relation to this publication may be liable to criminal prosecution and civil claims for damages.

The author has asserted his right to be identified as the author of this work in accordance with the Copyright, Designs and Patents Act 1988.

First published 2004 by
PALGRAVE MACMILLAN
Houndmills, Basingstoke, Hampshire RG21 6XS and
175 Fifth Avenue, New York, N.Y. 10010
Companies and representatives throughout the world

PALGRAVE MACMILLAN is the global academic imprint of the Palgrave Macmillan division of St. Martin's Press, LLC and of Palgrave Macmillan Ltd. Macmillan® is a registered trademark in the United States, United Kingdom and other countries. Palgrave is a registered trademark in the European Union and other countries.

ISBN 0–333–98083–2 paperback

This book is printed on paper suitable for recycling and made from fully managed and sustained forest sources.

A catalogue record for this book is available from the British Library.

10 9 8 7 6 5 4 3 2 1
13 12 11 10 09 08 07 06 05 04

Printed in China

Contents

List of figures

List of tables

Acknowledgements

Numerous people have given me their time and support in the writing of this work. In particular I would like to acknowledge the help received from all the patients and staff in the hospital, hospice, nursing home and residential settings I describe in this book. Their support was invaluable. I would also like to acknowledge the support from my family Marie, Joe, Rob and Ryan and my mentor and close friend who requested not to be acknowledged but for whom the words 'without his help' are entirely appropriate. Lastly, I dedicate this book to the memory of my parents, their passing inspired me to write about the experience of death and dying and taught me the importance of living for today.

Introduction

The provision of care for dying people in more contemporary terms is described as palliative care, although terminal care, hospice care and palliative care are used interchangeably to mean the same (Doyle 1994). Palliative care should not be associated exclusively with terminal care since many patients require palliative care often from the time of diagnosis. Terminal care is only one stage of palliative care and usually refers to the final stages of the person's life. Despite the different usages, it is generally recognised that palliative care is devoted to the care of people whose disease is no longer responsive to curative treatment (WHO 2002). As a relatively new emerging discipline palliative care is a dynamic and exciting field of work. It has helped to demystify our 'last taboo' – death and has been responsible for advances taking place in the control of pain and other distressing symptoms which have adversely affected the quality of terminal care. For over 30 years since the inception of the modern hospice movement, hospice care and the provision of palliative care more widely, has changed the face of modern nursing care both in and outside of institutions. The care of dying people has become much wider to include non-cancer diseases such as Acquired Immune Deficiency Syndrome (AIDS) and includes an examination of the psychosocial and spiritual dimensions of care with nurses becoming the major care providers. Currently the care of dying people takes place in a variety of different contexts, mainly hospitals where the majority of people die (Office of National Statistics (ONS 2000), hospices, where a small minority of deaths take place (Field & James 1993) and in community settings including the patient's home as well as a range of residential care settings such as elderly care homes. The focus of this book is the way in which different settings influence and shape the provision of care for the dying person and those who accompany them during the advanced stages of their illness.

The introduction represents a map of the book and explains the role of the author as researcher in each of the settings, hospital, hospice, community and home. It explains how each of the four parts to the book focuses on specific aspects of nursing care and also identifies the relevant literature and discusses some of the dominant theoretical frameworks which underpin our under-standing of death and dying in contemporary British society. Each chapter is fully referenced and contains a summary as well as a selection of useful further reading. The main focus of the book is the influence of the different contexts/environments on the quality of care for the dying person.

Part I comprises the first three chapters of the book and provides an account of my hospital research. It also contains a reflective chapter which examines the way in which nurses manage patients who are recovering in hospital and those who are dying. Each chapter focuses on similar issues relating to and raised by nursing dying patients in hospital, examining the influence of organisational culture and individual perceptions of care. Chapter 3 critically reviews the evidence from the hospital research and identifies tensions and positive attributes to the provision of effective care in a hospital context. As a whole, Part I provides a feel for the conditions in which hospital care takes place as well as allowing for an examination of some of the underlying features of terminal care in a hospital setting.

Part II describes hospice care and comprises Chapters 4 and 5. Chapter 4 describes the social and clinical management of dying patients informed by my research as a participant observer at The Beeches, a 12-bedded hospice. The chapter includes a brief overview of the origins and philosophy of the hospice movement, and gives an account of nurses' and patients' experiences in a hospice setting. Chapter 5 examines a number of ways to improve palliative care in hospitals through the use of Integrated Care Pathways (ICPs), Hospital Based Specialist Palliative Care Teams (HBSPCTs) and improved Multi-Disciplinary Team (MDT) working.

Part III consists of Chapters 6 and 7 and focuses attention onto the care of dying patients in the community. These chapters provide the reader with the opportunity of examining differences in the way terminal care is organised in community residential care establishments. An account is given of the care of residents in a nursing home (Cedar House) and a residential care establishment (Newlands). Despite sharing similar practices with hospital care, these institutions appear to have a more individual approach to the care of residents, a significant number of whom will have lived in the setting for many years. In Chapter 6, the author draws on a study of the day to day management of patients in a large nursing home. Interviews with nurses and health care support workers form the basis of the discussion about the pressures and challenges facing primary carers in non-hospital/hospice contexts. Contextual differences are discussed and comparative analysis made to highlight the issues associated with dying in non-hospital environments.

Part IV considers the many issues facing those who are dying at home and describes the experiences of patients and professionals dealing with cancer and non-cancer death in the community. Chapter 8 focuses on the challenges facing community nurses and examines the experience of families, who with nurses, share the terminal care of the dying person. Chapter 8 also includes an examination of the care of people dying at home together with my experiences of accompanying community nurses visiting terminally ill patients in their own homes. This chapter also includes an account of my family experience of caring for my dying Father. The final Chapter (9) considers the care of a dying person in a post-modern society and considers the type of terminal care provision given by families at the beginning of the 20th century so eloquently described by David Clark (2000). This final part of the book examines the debate concerning the preferences patients express for wanting to die in their own home (Seale 1991) and examines the rationale behind this. The final chapter compares and contrasts the problems, challenges and potential possibilities of institutional versus home death and provides an account of why dying at home may not always be in the patient's best interests.

Methodological considerations

The research data, underpinning much of the book, was collected whilst undertaking a doctoral study of the care of dying patients in hospital (Costello 2000). The research design was based on an ethnographic approach, and involved utilising a number of different research methods such as participant observation of nurses working in hospital wards and also by carrying out semi-structured interviews with doctors and nurses. The hospital study involved 150 hours of observation and took place in two different hospitals both of which focused on elderly care. The hospital research took two years to undertake and was completed at the end of 1998. The hospital study was supplemented by a further study of the care of dying patients in a new hospice (The Beeches), which had both in-patient and day hospice facilities. The hospice study was also based on an ethnographic design and adopted similar research methods, i.e. participant observation and interviews, in order to elicit details of working practices. The data from both the hospital and hospice studies form the basis of Parts I and II of the book.

The data for Parts III and IV, was derived from time spent shadowing district nurses and residential care – nursing home staff whilst going about their every day work with clients, both in their own homes and in residential care and nursing home settings. Observation of district nurses and residential and nursing home staff and clients formed the basis for the descriptions of care in a home; both in a residential care and nursing care home and the patient's own home. The penultimate chapter is focused on caring for dying patients in the community and includes as an illustration my experience of caring for my terminally ill Father, describing some of the practical and professional issues involved in end of life care from a personal perspective.

Theoretical assumptions

A number of concepts and theoretical frameworks are used to underpin the observations and accounts contained in the book, which adopts a largely sociological perspective. Most of our activities as nurses in the context of work are shaped by the patterns of interaction that take place between individuals and professional groups. These patterns or social structures are not random and are often highly structured and organised in a regular and repetitive way. Many social structures impinge on each other such as the delivery of the meal trolley, the cleaning routine, ward rounds and the involvement of members of the multi-disciplinary team. All these interactions may be seen as the infrastructure or framework, which underpins our working lives. Sociologists and others have commented on the importance of social structure and its influence on the world of work. In general I draw on the work of Berger & Luckman (1991) as well as structuralist theorists namely

Levi-Strauss (1968) and more recently Anthony Giddens (1997) particularly in relation to social structure and ideas about structuration theory. Philosophically, Levi-Strauss argues that the culture of a society provides a set of concepts for the construction of a sense of reality. Giddens (1997) extends the structuralist characterisation of theory to incorporate an interrelation between structure and action. Structure can be both enabling and constraining and is seen as any social arrangement such as the roles doctors, nurses and other health care workers occupy within a given context. The rules and conventions I refer to in the early chapters, which help to shape actions, may be regarded as *deep structures* which in themselves have responsibility for the production of a surface structure. An illustration of this is 'curtaining off', drawing the curtains around hospital beds when a deceased patient is taken to the mortuary. This helps to keep death hidden through a process of sequestration attempting to (but often failing), to hide death away from the living. Another example is the medical ward round where a series of actions and roles are played out within the public forum of the hospital ward. The ward round may be seen as a structure which enables patients' cases to be reviewed and often involves decisions being made to discharge patients or review medication, thereby enabling patient treatments to be determined as well as 'freeing up' beds. Conversely, many nurses put a great deal of effort into the management of the ward round and often if ward rounds are formally organised they can put constraints on other activities such as attending other departments for investigations.

Throughout the book I make use of the concept of structure and agency (as the two main determinants of social outcome) to make sense of the relationship between what nurses do and the structural constraints they are faced with. Agency refers to the power of individual 'actors' to operate independently of the determining constraints of social structure. The term is often used to convey the volitional and purposive nature of human activity, which is in itself opposed to the constrained determined aspects imposed by structure. Structure and agency are terms used more widely in sociology from ethnomethodology, phenomenology and symbolic interactionism. In many ways individual 'actors' are characterised as supporters of the structure as well as playing a part in its development. In this sense the more traditional view of the

nurse as the compliant servant carrying out the doctors orders
produces an image of nurses as *cultural dopes*. This stereotypical
view is not one I share since my observations lead me to conclude
that nurses play an active if not disproportionate role in con-
structing their own reality within the culture of the hospital ward.
Giddens argues however that individuals play a clear role in determining outcomes, acting more as *mediums* than what others refer
to as *cultural dopes*. Berger & Luckman (1991) in a macro sense,
point out that the relationship between structure and agency is
one whereby society forms the individual, who then creates society in a continuous dialectic. For Berger & Luckman (1991:121),
the social construction of reality involves an understanding of
structure and agency and the need to create institutional order,
for them:

> The legitimation of the institutional order is also faced with
> the ongoing necessity of keeping chaos at bay. All social real-
> ity is precarious and all societies are constructions in the face
> of chaos.

Berger & Luckman and others (Bhaskar 1979) use social
constructionism to highlight the view that it is the interrelationship between structure and agency that gives rise to much social
action, asserting that this helps to control chaos by the imposition
of order. Needless to say there is little consensus about the exact
nature of the relationship between structure and agency as well as
there being much debate about what constitutes structure. It is
generally considered that structure and agency do have a complementary relationship despite the diversity of opinion on this issue.

In relation to my observations of hospital wards described in
the first three chapters, I examine the social structure and in particular how rules and routine play an essential part in the provision of care. The argument is advanced that hospitals as institutions,
exercise a significant amount of control over death and the dying
patient, largely through medical dominance which often involved
conflict between doctors and nurses (arising from issues related to
ethical dilemmas such as documenting Do Not Resuscitate (DNR)
orders). The outcomes arising from discourse between nurses and
doctors are a collective construction of a *controlling culture* replete
with rules and expectations for patients as well as doctors and

nurses. The context in which this rule construction takes place serves to reinforce and perpetuate control. Patients are expected to observe rules such as not asking too many questions, being compliant and following instructions. These constructions help to maintain the sentimental order of the ward and are themselves constructed by doctors and nurses as a form of control to ensure the containment of chaos. In Chapters 6 and 7, I describe the care in non-hospital/hospice settings which demonstrate contrasting features as well as similarities with the institutional hospital routines, such as meal times and drug administration. There is also a clear lack of hierarchical domination between professional groups. This demarcates the contexts and where there are fewer professional groups, there appear to be more opportunities for individual agents to be creative in defining their care culture. The absence of explicit hierarchy or the 'low profile' adopted by medical staff in hospices (Chapter 4) also has an enabling effect in allowing nurses to become more patient focused and for the patients' individual needs to be paid greater attention. In Part III of the book the nursing home and residential care home settings demonstrate a lack of medical dominance and fewer powerful figures to take part in the construction of a controlling culture. In these settings, there are vestiges of the type of institutional care found in hospitals (in terms of the rigidity of the routine), although this often appears to be influenced by the needs of the elderly residents as much as the needs of the staff. Non-hospital settings tended to be more liberal and patient focused in terms of the way in which the needs of the institution take second place to those of the patient. There is also evidence that residents are able to 'claim back control' and appeal to rules in non-hospital contexts. The way professional caregivers in all contexts provide care for dying patients is linked with the organisational culture and the way in which the culture is influenced and controlled by those with most power. Ultimately the construction of a culture of care is influenced by the context in which that care takes place, which in itself brings one back to the relationship between structure and agency. Nurses in hospital can become empowered to change the structures that constrain them from doing what they believe to be things to improve patient care such as spending more time with them, although this may be different from what the patient wants or needs.

Key issues in the provision of care for dying patients

Despite the proliferation of palliative care services and the improvements made, there are a number of notable challenges facing palliative care practitioners. Historically at least, it is clear as Wilkes (1993) points out that the hospice movement in general and palliative care in particular has been responsible for bringing about improvements in the standards of care for dying people. Palliative care has been recognised as a fluid concept, which is also context and culture bound (Abu-Saad 2001 : 134). Despite the rapid and often radical improvements in care for dying patients, there remain a number of challenges for the current and future provision of high standards of care. These may be seen as; the medicalisation of death and dying, issues to do with access and provision of palliative care, quality of life assessment, communication and multi-disciplinary teamwork.

Medicalisation

The emergence of palliative medicine as a sub specialty in 1987 is seen by many as an indication of increased biomedical influences on the care of dying patients (Biswas 1993, Field 1994, Clark & Seymour 1999). A number of writers have raised issues concerning the direction that palliative care is going. A number have asked questions about the emphasis on the increasing influence of biomedical approaches made towards palliating the symptoms of diseases such as cancer (Corner & Dunlop 1997, Clark & Seymour 1999, Clark 2002, Thomas 2003). The medicalisation of death and dying is seen to be taking place partly because of the merger between mainstream care and palliative care. It is also apparent as Clark & Seymour (1999:105) point out that palliative care is being drawn into:

> The pervasive development of a form of 'therapeutic' culture in which the universal experience of suffering is brought into the remit of professional health and re-characterised as a 'problem' with a medical solution.

Citing the work of Cassell (1991), Clark & Seymour (1999) point out that a person's self identity is bound up with their experience of illness. The 'making medical' of a person's dying trajectory which includes experiencing suffering as part of a process dominated by biomedical influences and leading to a disempowerment of the patient. The medicalisation thesis much debated in the last decade has resonance today as the hospice movement and palliative care practice spreads into non-traditional areas such as nursing homes and residential care settings. It is also clear that medicalisation involves nurses and others who play a part in patient surveillance and monitoring. This takes the form of a subjectification of the patient experience (May 1992) whereby nurses are encouraged to engage in meaningful relationships often through the use of techniques such as counselling with patients, in order to ensure that care meets the criteria for becoming holistic. The notion of holism is disingenuous in the sense that relationships with the patient are unbalanced in terms of power and subject to the many organisational pressures for patients to conform to the needs of the organisation and its routines (Lupton 1995, James & Field 1996).

Lupton (1995) and others (Hunt 1991, May 1992) point out that nurses' attempts to subjectify patients' experiences through the use of informality, conversation and attempts to engage in counselling discourses may also form part of patient surveillance, which may be seen as an integral part of medicalisation. The organisational processes which together demonstrate evidence of medicalisation are not isolated to medical practice and more recently have been influenced by the work of nurses and others who have played a key role in medicalisation of the patients' palliative care experiences.

Throughout the book it is stressed that dying is a normal process that takes place in a variety of settings. It is however made clear that in certain settings such as hospitals where the most criticisms are made, dying can be problematic and unpleasant for the patient and the family. Some hospitals retain traditional monolithic and autocratic attitudes whereby the needs of the organisation take priority and become more important than those whom they set out to serve. This dominant feature of many larger hospitals may be seen as part of the problem of why some patients and families reflect on their experiences as a bad death, leaving them an often unhappy and distressing legacy about the loss of a loved one. It is perhaps in hospital where many of the practices exist (and where most people die) that it can be said to be medicalised and ultimately disempowers patients. Other settings demonstrate similar problems, although the evidence suggests that hospitals and their staff have numerous problematic issues to do with power struggles between different professional groups (Porter 1991). The context in which death takes place helps to shape the patient's ability to feel part of what is going on rather than where practices are highly medicalised, and patients become passive recipients of care as a result of the prevailing practices adopted by those who control and wield the power.

Access and provision

Despite the many improvements in treatment and the raised standards of care resulting from the provision of palliative and hospice services, the care received by dying patients in hospices and specialist palliative care centres is not without criticism. In particular, questions have been raised regarding the elitist nature of palliative care for focusing on the needs of the few, particularly those fortunate enough to be able to obtain a hospice bed (Douglas 1992, Clark 1993, Walter 1999). Hospices themselves have developed a reputation for exclusivity although in the last decade this has changed with attention focused on a range of people with non-malignant conditions such as Multiple Sclerosis (MS), Motor Neurone Disease (MND) and HIV and AIDS. The issue of access and provision of palliative care has also been extended to people from black and ethnic minority groups in terms of improving access and to assess the culture specific palliative care needs of these patients (NCHSPCS 1995, Diver et al 2003).

A number of influencing factors seem to shape the access and provision of palliative care services. The first may be the lack of an accurate definition of what palliative care is. Despite the now well known WHO (1990) definition, the terminology used in palliative care seems to expand the boundaries and be rather more inclusive than previous attempts at definition. Another consideration is funding. Many voluntary hospices founded on charters which specified that hospice services be provided for cancer patients, struggle to provide access to non-cancer patients, but do accept patients with non-cancer conditions such as MS and MND, and perhaps less often those with AIDS. The lack of attention given to those who are not considered 'first choice' for palliative care services has influenced others to consider people in this position as the 'disadvantaged dying' (Addington-Hall et al 1998). The palliative care needs of patients with non-malignant disease have been highlighted in the NCHSPCS (1998) guidelines *Reaching Out* which indicate that:

> The palliative care approach aims to promote both physical and psychosocial well being. It is a vital and integral part of all clinical practice, whatever the illness or its stage. (NCHSPCS 1998:12)

There are a number of possible reasons and factors involved in why there might be reluctance to widen access and provision to palliative care services. Some writers have identified that the diagnosis of a non-malignant condition causes less distress to patients and that families and patients accept the symptoms as inevitable (Addington-Hall & Higginson 2001). There are also issues related to how to categorise the stages of a non-malignant disease and when the terminal stages begin. One prospective hospital study carried out in 1988 included patients dying from non-malignant disease:

> highlighted certain problems such as nausea, anorexia and pressure sores in this group. It was found that moderate and severe pain occurred as often in these patients as in patients with cancer (Hockley et al 1988:1716).

Since the publication of the *Reaching Out* guidelines more evidence and debate about the needs of people with non-malignant disease has taken place, although there is relatively little empirical research that matches studies conducted with cancer patients.

Quality of life

Debates about quality of life are at the centre of palliative care ideology. Indeed palliative care in providing a new ethic for the care of dying patients has focused most of its attention upon finding ways for improving quality of life. It is useful to remind

ourselves that as a discipline, palliative care arose out of concern
for improving pain control and management of distressing symptoms, as well as scepticism over medical intervention and a need
to respond to health care consumerism. These have all played a
part in helping to shape the way in which palliative care is developed today. The National Council for Hospice and Specialist
Palliative Care Services (NCHSPCS 1997), identifies that the
defining characteristics of a specialist palliative care service include
the existence of a quality assurance programme used to review
practice as well as clinical audit tools and a research programme.
The search for quality particularly in the 1990s has gained promi-
nence through palliative care. Whilst not only improving the quality of life, the World Health Organisation includes in its definition,
that palliative care sets out to prevent complications, seeks to
relieve suffering and positively influence the course of the patient's
illness (WHO 2002). Numerous ways of measuring quality of life
have been used although as Aspinall et al (2003) in a review of
the literature on using satisfaction to measure quality conclude,
that the current use of satisfaction to measure quality in palliative care is seriously flawed due to its prescriptive nature, lack of
definition and a lack of conceptual clarity. However, there is a
tension here between the growing desire of many agencies for
example Macmillan Cancer Relief, who are very keen to develop
the notion of 'user involvement' and to ask cancer patients what
they perceive satisfaction to be. Aspinall et al (2003) point out
that there are few alternatives to asking patients and suggest that
'snap shot images' of satisfaction are transitory and unreliable as
a way of ensuring that the user's perceptions of quality of life are
amplified. Measuring quality of health care, although difficult, is
an important way of developing future services.

Communication and multi-disciplinary teamworking

Multi-disciplinary teamwork has been consistently important in
the care of dying patients judging by the references made to this
form of communication in policy documents, *NHS Community
Care Act* (Department of Health 1990), *The New NHS: Modern,
Dependable* (Department of Health 1997), *The Cancer Plan*
(Department of Health 2000). Reports such as the Calman &
Hine (1995) specifically identify multi-professional teams as

forums for the delivery of flexible and individualised care contributing towards a more comprehensive service.

A number of influences impinge on effective palliative care provision with the most pervasive being intra-professional communication particularly between members of the multi-disciplinary team. Nurses make a major contribution to the success of the MDT largely because they become the patient's continuous care-giver and form the nucleus of the team (Carson et al 1997, Hill 1998). The literature relating to the organisation and delivery of services to patients with a range of cancer and non-cancer conditions is replete with problems and challenges in being able to meet the specific needs of the patient, particularly relating to information giving and providing access to specialist services (Davidson et al 1995, Luker et al 1996). Moreover problems have been identified with the development of effective communication between professionals and recipients of care (Fallowfield 1995, Wilkinson & Mula 2003). There is a clear view that the role of the MDT is to support and advise patients and their families in order to provide good symptom control, share information and give essential psychosocial support. Key players in this are the medical consultant's team, nursing staff, the GP and a host of primary care and hospital staff. An effective MDT can assist in co-coordinating care between existing services as well as facilitating admission to and discharge from hospital. By liaising with community staff, MDT support can also enable respite care to be provided; as well as putting patients and families in touch with essential medical and nursing services such as Macmillan nurses in and out of the hospital setting (Irvine 1993). Multi-disciplinary teamwork harnesses the skills required for the task and combines them in a unique way in order to increase services, reduce individual workloads, enhance collegial support and provide cross fertilisation of ideas (Ovretveit 1995).

The ability of the MDT to bring about effective communication is related to the way in which each of the individuals in the team communicates. In some cases, power differentials between doctors and nurses can limit team functioning (Costello 1994). In other cases the hierarchical nature of organisational culture within the hospital can impede effective teamwork and lead to fragmentation (Soothill et al 1995, Luker et al 2002). The work of the MDT is often complex in terms of membership, role expectation and the relationship between the individuals involved. Some teams work well through a process of compliance to each other's perceived abilities, other teams may not function well due to difficulties in understanding their specific role as a group or because they lack the necessary resources and support enabling them to make a full contribution to teamworking (Luker et al 2002). Despite MDTs being seen as an effective forum for delivering care, the evidence suggests that optimal team functioning is difficult to achieve (Hill 1998). Hill found that although teamworking was highly valued within a hospital palliative care team, the internal dynamics of the team in terms of role blurring and role ambiguity prevented the type of cohesion taking place that may have led to improvements in service delivery.

The conditions under which all health care professionals work, the structures, roles and regulations one helps to construct also have an impact on the recipients of care and treatment. The context in which care takes place helps to shape working practices as all the chapters will demonstrate. The actions of doctors, nurses, health support workers, allied professionals and patients are linked to and complement the care setting. The culture of care is a reflection of the mosaic found within the particular context be it a hospital, hospice or other care setting where residents are approaching the end of their lives.

Institutions that care for the sick and dying such as hospitals have long been conceived of as social systems which function because of those who play a part in their construction – the staff and the residents. It is well known that the effects of life in institutions can have a marked effect on patients and staff (Goffman 1968, Miller & Gwynne 1972). The context is clearly influenced by the way in which patients recovering from illness are cared for in the same setting as those who are dying. Collectively, Part I provides a feel for the environment in which hospital care takes place as well as identifying some of the key issues in shaping care of dying patients in the hospital context.

Part I will now turn our attention to the hospital setting. What follows is an account of the care and treatment of patients in three elderly care wards. The chapter will consider the way care is organised and provided for patients who are living with chronic illness and those who are dying.

Part I
Caring in a hospital context

Part I provides an account of my hospital research and contains a reflective chapter which examines the way in which nurses manage patients who are recovering in hospital and those who are dying. Each chapter focuses on similar issues relating to and raised by nursing dying patients in hospital, examining the influence of organisational culture and individual perceptions of care. Chapter 3 critically reviews the evidence from the hospital research and identifies tensions and positive attributes to the provision of effective care in a hospital context. As a whole, Part I provides a feel for the conditions in which hospital care takes place as well as allowing for an examination of some of the underlying features of terminal care in a hospital setting.

1 Nursing the dying in hospital: the challenge to care

Introduction

This chapter focuses on the way in which death and dying are managed in different hospital settings and examines some of the experiences faced by a range of patients and staff in different contexts. The aim of the chapter is to critically review the origins of hospital care, examining the problems and challenges facing nurses and doctors who work in environments that are not conducive to terminal care, but where death is all too familiar. The chapter will consider the key areas where death regularly takes place and highlight the challenges facing nurses caring for patients with a variety of different medical conditions. Reflective incidents are used to describe scenarios illustrating the complexity of death and dying in diverse areas such as the Accident and Emergency department (A&E), elderly care wards and Intensive Care Units (ICUs). The death of a baby in A&E and in a maternity unit is contrasted with the death of a young woman in ICU and an older person in an elderly care unit. All the deaths, although sad, reflect social attitudes about death and dying; revealing that age is an important factor influencing the way nurses respond when a person dies. By examining the context in which patients die in hospital, the reader can see how differing hospital contexts help to shape expectations about dying and also make a difference to the way professional staff behave when a person dies.

The origins of hospital care

Despite the shift from hospital to community care seen in the 1990s, by far the majority of people still die in institutions, primarily hospitals (Field & James 1993, Costello 2000). Despite home being the preferred place of death the majority die in institutions with one quarter of all hospital beds being taken up by patients in the last year of life (Higginson et al 1998). Historically, the death of a person in hospital, especially when the institution originated from a workhouse, was often viewed in a derogatory way with some older people believing that if they went into hospital they would never come out alive. Although for some, this was sadly true, more recently increasing numbers of people are discharged following a short period of hospitalisation and make a full recovery at home.

Originally, hospitals were not designed to care specifically for the dying, and many are more suitable for managing situations in which the patient gets better and then goes home. This curative ideology has permeated the philosophy of many doctors and nurses and may be seen as one of the motivating factors 'in the push' towards improvements in medical technology. Unfortunately, many people admitted to hospital, particularly older people, have numerous medical problems and despite improvements in health care and medical technology, the care they require may not always be based on cure. Care should be aimed at improving the quality of life by adopting and implementing palliative care principles. From within this paradoxical situation, where cure is the aim of doctors and nurses, rather than caring, the social process of dying in hospital is examined.

What's wrong with hospitals?

Hospitals have rarely occupied a popular public image and as the history of voluntary hospitals portrays, patients were also not highly regarded. Cohen (1964:20) points out that patients in voluntary hospitals were regarded as:

> Miserable objects of charity who were severely disciplined for minor infringements of hospital rules.

In the London Hospital anyone found complaining about treatment was disqualified from further attention. Other hospitals imposed strict regulations about swearing, gaming or drinking, and lights out by 20.00 hours. At Guy's Hospital anyone found smoking was immediately discharged.

Since its inception in 1948, the National Health Service (NHS) has sought to provide high quality care for all its patients irrespective of their means, creed or medical condition. The history of many British NHS hospitals is one replete with evidence of staff shortages and facilities and peppered with numerous scandals about lack of care and patient neglect. May (1995:85) has pointed out that:

> The organisation of the general hospital is profoundly hostile to the expression of the patient's deepest emotions.

More recently media constructions and public perceptions of hospital care have been shaped by bed crises, a term which has been ushered into common parlance in the last decade. What may be argued to be lacking in hospitals is the personal touch and individuality afforded to people in their home environment. Mills et al's (1994) study of 13 wards found that there was evidence of neglect and poor standards of terminal care being provided to dying patients. Despite the poor history of care for the dying patient in hospital, the care of dying patients has often been seen as an important part of hospital care and treatment as *The NHS Cancer Plan* (Department of Health 2000) points out:

> Providing the best possible care for dying patients remains of paramount importance. Too many patients still experience distressing symptoms, poor nursing care, poor psychological and social support and inadequate communication from healthcare professionals during the final stages of an illness.

This part of the book considers the experience of dying in hospital and looks closely at some of the key issues surrounding hospital death including: lack of individual care; the management of dying patients in a variety of contexts; and the challenges facing doctors and nurses in providing terminal care within a curative environment not designed to meet the needs of the dying and their family. Despite the negative connotations of NHS treatment, as well as the preferences for people to die at home (Seale & Cartwright 1994), many people find comfort in the fact that hospitals offer security and are generally considered to be safe environments to occupy when ill. A significant number of people find it impossible to care for their dying family member at home and for many others death at home is not a preferred or viable option. Hospital care offers the security of knowing professional help is on hand, together with a degree of social contact with others. The security of having physical needs for warmth, shelter, protection and social contact met within an environment where doctors and nurses are available 24 hours a day, appeals to many vulnerable patients, such as older people, who may not have carers available at home who can meet their particular needs.

Processing patients: the warehousing model of care

Hospitals, particularly psychiatric institutions, have received much attention from social scientists, sociologists and others in relation to the impact that such organisations have on those who reside in them. It is clear from the literature that treatment of illness is only one part of a hospital's function. The relationship between the professional care provider and the care recipient also forms part of the patient's trajectory, as well as the relationship between the patient and the organisation. Many traditional writers conceive of the hospital as a social system functioning in an environment, a system that is created and maintained by patients and staff alike (Etzioni 1964, Goffman 1968, Miller & Gwynne 1972). Some of the features of institutional life reflect surviving in a setting that depersonalises the 'inmate' and causes them to learn patterns of behaviour and subservience which more accurately reflect the needs of the organisation not the individual. The following anonymous poem called *Rapid Access and Me* was written by an out-patient and illustrates the patient's sense of subservience:

Rapid Access and Me
I have been booked in the clinic and I have been taken to a
    room,
I am asked to strip from the waist upwards and the con-
    sultant will be in soon,
I am sat on the edge of the bed my heart all of a flutter,
In comes the consultant and I start to stutter,
Many questions are asked and lots of answers returned,
I look at the consultant and wonder what he has learned.

The attitudes and ideology of hospital staff play a significant role in shaping the approaches nurses and doctors make towards treatment and care. Miller & Gywnne (1972) discuss two models of care that take place in residential settings making reference to hospital based care. Warehousing is a term used to describe care based on a need to prolong physical life by enabling the patient to develop a greater sense (and practice) of dependency of the care of elderly patients on the professional caregiver. Baker (1978) used the term to describe her findings in an elderly care hospital. Today nurses use the term 'sheep dipping' to describe situations when physical care is prioritised above all else due to a range of organisational constraints (largely due to staffing problems). The patient's role in this model is to develop a dependency and have their role defined. Any attempt by patients to break out of their institutional role prevents the warehousing process from working effectively. Hospital residents are therefore encouraged to be 'good patients' in terms of their physical problems. The process works well if the patient accepts their situation and acts in a compliant manner. An example of the types of sanctions used to ensure compliance are labelling, illustrated in a psychiatric context by Johnson (1993).

In contrast, the horticultural model is based on encouraging independence in the patient who has a number of unfulfilled capacities. The professional's role in this model is to develop the patient's capacities. The thrust of this progressive approach is to rehabilitate the patient in the belief that he/she is capable of becoming more effective and independent. The nurse's role is to help the patient by nurturance of strengths and to provide opportunities for personal growth.

Both models of care are not without their weaknesses. The warehousing model is inhumane and has obvious inadequacies. These include lack of attention to patients' physical and emotional needs and the reinforcement of patients' problems at the same time highlighting the needs of the organisation as being of greater importance. Having said that, acceptance of dependency may suit some more than others and depends much on the stage in their illness. Terminally ill patients need physical care but also recognition of the many psychosocial needs which can arise at the end of life.

The horticultural model with its obvious idealistic appeal is however flawed in terms of seeing people as being more than their physical difficulties, especially when the person is terminally ill or in some cases unable to be rehabilitated, for example those with profound MS or MND. For some, accepting the loss of their personal freedoms may be a small price to pay for receiving effective skilled physical care, which may be their priority and suit their needs better than attempts at providing psychological care. The person with MS or MND may feel as disempowered in a context utilising the horticultural mode, as the relatively healthy young counterpart with cancer cared for using a warehousing model.

Dying in acute care contexts: a matter of life and death

It may be argued that few are ever prepared for the death of a loved one and when faced with the loss, it can still come as a shock. Within hospitals, deaths can and do happen unexpectedly and present a number of challenges for hospital staff, particularly those working in acute areas such as the operating theatres, A&E departments, ICUs, and Coronary Care Units (CCUs). In these areas, designed to save life and improve the quality of that life, death may be felt as a sense of failure, particularly if the patient is a child or if the staff experience a sense of guilt because it was possible to save them 'if only' circumstances had been different. Describing the unexpected death of patients in A&E departments, Wright (1996) points out that sudden death is one of the most traumatic crisis events that can be experienced by both patients and hospital staff. Not only is the death of a patient a major source of distress, also the subsequent bereavement of the family can reduce their coping abilities, leaving an emotional scar that may be felt for the rest of their lives.

Reflective incident

Karen (Staff Nurse) was on a late duty in A&E when a young couple came in carrying a baby wrapped up in a blanket. Bypassing the usual formalities they were ushered into a cubicle and were seen immediately by a doctor. The baby (7 months old) was very pale and still, Karen could see that it was not breathing. The parents were en route to visit friends and although the baby was asleep, the mother Zoë sensed there was something wrong. They stopped the car and found that baby Matthew was not breathing and drove straight to the hospital, a 10-minute drive away. Karen had never seen a dead baby before:

> I will never forget the look on the mother's face when the
> doctor said 'I'm sorry I'm afraid there is nothing we can do
> for him', I felt angry, very, very sad and upset, I didn't really
> know how to react. I was angry at the doctor for not making
> it sound more positive, but also I was angry at myself. I also
> felt very useless, all this technology and expertise, all this power
> and yet we couldn't do a thing for the baby, I will never for-
> get their faces, their shock and sadness. I realised I should
> have been more professional, but I cried with the parents who
> were roughly the same age as me, it was as if I shared their
> sadness, I became a casualty that night, it was awful.

The emotional trauma associated with sudden death is often experienced by both staff and patients alike, challenging the professionals to not only manage the anxiety of others, but also to cope
with their own anguish. Reflecting on this incident with the baby,
some may be critical of the staff nurse who could perhaps have
remained in control of her feelings in order to offer support to
the traumatised parents. However in some cases it can be com-
forting for recipients of care to be able to see the human side of
'the professionals' and a greater sense of security can be gained
from knowing that the experts are also human. How nurses and
doctors react in such situations depends on the particular circumstances, previous experience and the way they are feeling at
the time. Jolley & Brykczynska (1992) point out that expressing
the way we feel as nurses and having the courage to show our
sensitivity and become aware of our own vulnerability, can help us
to stay in touch with our sense of compassion. Much depends
however on the climate in which we work, the supportive nature
of those around us and the extent to which hospital staff are able
to feel supported when dealing with traumatic circumstances, a
topic which will be further discussed later in the chapter.

Death and dying in maternity/paediatric care units

The birth of a baby is one of the happiest moments in our lives,
which makes the death of a baby one of the most tragic events

that we may experience. In the Middle Ages, when the death of a child was more commonplace, as it still is today in certain developing countries, the death of a child caused relatively little disruption to the community in which it lived (Aries 1974). Today, the death of a baby at or shortly after birth gives rise to personal crisis and an extreme form of grief, which often requires sensitive professional support in order to make sense of what many regard as a family tragedy. The hospital staff in maternity units share in both the joy of birth and the grief of mothers whose babies are stillborn (born after 24 weeks gestation, and show no signs of life) as well as perinatal deaths (stillbirths and those who die within the first 7 days of life, irrespective of gestation time). Special Care Baby Units (SCBUs) often admit babies who are born premature (before 28 weeks gestation) and die within the first 28 days of life, who are referred to as neonatal deaths. Stewart & Dent (1994:54) point out that medical terminology used at the time of stillbirth can have a profound effect on parents; terms such as foetal distress, in lay terms can be perceived as an implication that the baby has experienced pain and discomfort.

Reflective incident

Susan (24 years old) was expecting her first baby and throughout pregnancy had been experiencing blood pressure problems, but despite close monitoring by her community midwife was admitted 3 weeks before term to the antenatal unit for rest and observation. Subsequently during labour Susan experienced problems and the baby became distressed necessitating an emergency caesarean section. Despite the maternity team working as quickly as possible, the baby was born alive but died in the labour room after a few minutes. The news was broken to Susan and her partner Alan in the side room, once Susan had fully recovered from the anaesthetic. They were both devastated:

> It's like your worst nightmare... I worried about something happening to the baby and something going wrong but not this, not this, it's just so unfair and wrong, we were going to be so happy.

The maternity staff were also devastated and the atmosphere in the unit was palpable with sadness. Susan's parents arrived and asked for the hospital priest. Susan and Alan were given time with the baby and a staff midwife waited outside the room. Alan took a photograph of the baby boy whom they called Edward after Susan's grandfather, who died the previous year. A piece of hair was taken from the baby and later that morning a short religious service took place in the hospital chapel. The maternity staff arranged for a handprint to be made of baby Edward. The Co-op funeral services came to pick up the baby and took him to the chapel of rest. Susan stayed in hospital for three days to recover from the surgery and was discharged home on the fourth day. The following day the funeral took place at the local Catholic Church with an abundance of flowers and mourners. Susan's parents arranged for the funeral party to take place at their house. The cost of the funeral was minimal because of the baby's age, the Co-op played a role in helping Susan and Alan consider Edward's death as a major loss, sending the family a memorial card after the funeral with a picture of Edward. One of the staff midwives who attended the delivery represented the hospital at the funeral. Two weeks after the funeral, the unit social worker rang Susan and Alan and asked if there was anything they could do. Susan had already contacted The Compassionate Friends (TCF) who provided bereavement advice and support. (See Useful contacts section)

The death of a child in our culture is a tragic event that challenges everyone involved with the family, in attempting to help the parents and other family members come to terms with their loss. Some parents feel a sense of comfort in not wanting to come to terms with the loss, rather appearing to want to feel the full impact of the death by embracing death and experiencing the full brunt of their loss. Others may appear to block out, deny or consider anything but the loss, as their way of coping. Sometimes these two extremes can cause conflict when they are experienced by people in the same family or by the parents themselves. Hindmarch (2000:34) points out:

> Whether personally or professionally involved, the death of a child is seen as the most difficult loss to cope with…to talk about and anticipate.

In hospital settings, where staff and families often share the same sense of impotence when coping with the death of a child, Hindmarch (2000:81) suggests that good practice involves the following:

- Be sensitive to the parent's needs.
- Avoid platitudes and statements that imply criticism of the child's care.
- Be prepared to listen: share feelings and memories.
- Do not give up visiting the family for fear of intruding (unless they request no visiting).
- Familiarise yourself with hospital procedures regarding police, funeral arrangements, social workers, chaplains and national bereavement resources.
- Be there for all the family, including siblings and grandparents.

As a professional staff member, it is always useful to know and be familiar with support agencies such as the Foundation for Sudden Infant Death (FSID) as well as TCF, a Quaker group who carry out invaluable bereavement support for families facing and dealing with loss. (see Useful contacts section) Richies & Dawson's (2000) research into family responses to death, highlights the need for professionals to appreciate both the complexity and diversity of grief reactions. They reinforce the need for doctors and nurses to be sensitive to the difficulties faced by families, as many individuals in the family experience the impact of loss in a different way. This they argue is a major challenge to the skills of the medical and nursing practitioners.

Death and dying in critical care contexts

Death in critical care areas such as ICU, CCU and High Dependency Units (HDUs) often takes place following attempts by doctors and nurses to 'save' the patient's life; numerous interventions are employed, notably the use of life preserving technology such as ventilators, in order to both extend life and improve its quality. Death in this context therefore carries with it enormous distress and sadness for the patient's family, along with numerous challenges and frustrations for staff working in situations of crisis. Many people would agree that areas such as CCU and ICU are places in which life saving measures become routine and the use of 'heroic' emergency measures add to the 'mystique' of these areas. Media portrayals such as *ER* and *Casualty* depict a glamorous image of doctors and nurses making life and death decisions, almost by the hour. Many would argue that in large critical care settings such as ICU, these media images are not far from the truth. There is also evidence that the glamorous image of 'high tech' areas is the reason why nurses find such places attractive areas in which to work, especially when compared to the comparatively mundane general medical, surgical and elderly care wards (Baker 1978). Despite their attraction as glamorous places in which to work, situations arise in ICU that create tremendous stress for staff, patients and relatives alike (Vachon 1987). In many cases ICUs record higher numbers of deaths per month compared with other hospital areas. Often staff turnover rates are much higher, partly because of the nature of the work, staff : patient ratios as well as the increasing amounts of stress experienced by nurses and doctors when staffing falls below optimum levels. When situations like this occur, managers often find that sickness-absence increases, giving rise to additional stress experienced by some nurses. Harry is a Senior Nurse managing one of the biggest and busiest ICUs in the country with a large complement of nurses; he finds it very frustrating when staffing levels mean nurses not only have to work harder, but also stress levels increase:

> When patient dependency and staffing resources do not correlate the increase in workload results in higher levels of stress within the unit. When we are full and there are some very complicated cases this can have a very adverse effect on the staff as a whole.

Mary Vachon (1987), a Canadian Nurse who has written extensively about the effects of terminal care and death in critical care areas, argues that staff stress and burn-out occur frequently in intensive care areas as a result of the high number of patients facing impending death and the complex and often very personal decisions made, concerning end of life issues.

Reflective incident

Kim was a 23 year old lady who was brutally attacked and raped by a man outside a nightclub in Manchester. She was brought into the A&E department unconscious, in a state of shock and with severe breathing difficulties as a result of her attack. She was transferred from the A&E department and attached to a ventilator in ICU. Neurological investigations revealed that she had in fact suffered damage to her brain stem as a result of the assault. Kim was unable to breathe unaided and if she were to be taken off the ventilator it seemed clear that she would imminently die. The hospital neurologist diagnosed her as being in a Persistent Vegetative State (PVS). Her attacker was apprehended by the police and was in custody having been charged with the assault, which he admitted to the police. Despite verifying Kim's condition with another neurologist together with two physicians and an anaesthetist, Kim's parents and immediate family could not come to terms with the diagnosis and prognosis and believed that she would one day regain consciousness. Their distress was compounded by a number of pressures placed on the medical staff to come to an early decision about taking Kim off the ventilator and allowing her to die with dignity. Kim's assailant was awaiting trial and likely to be charged with murder or manslaughter. Any decision to take Kim off the ventilator would result in death and would in legal terms reduce the possible charge to manslaughter. The hospital was informed that on no account could Kim be taken off the ventilator because of the legal implications involved in charging the assailant. The trial therefore did not take place for several months.

The family were offered counselling by the hospital, but declined. Kim's parents, her brother and sister, overwhelmed by grief, refused to accept the inevitability that she was going to die and had to experience a very traumatic period observing her in this state. Patients who are unable to communicate effectively with others when they are dying are said to be experiencing social death (Sweeting & Gilhooley 1991). This rather strange and distressing phenomenon related to a loss of personhood, renders the individual outside the normal boundaries of social contact, remaining in what Van Gennep (1972) refers to as '*a liminal state*'. The staff on the unit experienced tremendous stress as a result of the traumatic situation that prevailed. Many of the staff experienced personal distress, which was compounded by the problem of having to face the family on a regular basis and help them make sense of what was occurring at a very traumatic time. Kim was being cared for with great sensitivity, she received intravenous fluids and full monitoring. The family insisted on spending most of the day with her, returning the next morning. Sadly the situation deteriorated and Kim was removed from the ventilator the day before the case went to trial. At their request, the family was present when Kim was extubated and she died shortly afterwards. Arrangements had been made for Kim to be taken to the chapel of rest in order to bypass the mortuary. The family had previously planned the funeral arrangements and members of the ICU attended, as they had become very close to Kim and the rest of the family. Eventually Kim's assailant was found guilty of manslaughter and received a 10-year prison sentence.

Kim's death was a sad event, but also a great source of relief for both the family and the staff who shared the anticipatory grief (Costello 1999) of knowing 5 months earlier that death would take place. During this time adaptation to the death had taken place and many of the so-called 'stages of grieving' had been reached. Anticipatory grief is the affective experiences people undergo when they are aware that they are dying, with often the patient and their loved ones adapting to the impending loss and sharing similar reactions. Anticipatory grief may enable some people to prepare for the loss by adapting to the death, although as Rando (1986) has pointed out, the length of time spent awaiting death can sometimes have a detrimental effect on the soon-to-become-bereaved, especially if a child is involved.

Reflecting on Kim's situation, which was taken from a real hospital experience, there are a number of features of her death, which reveal insights into death and dying in hospital. First is the management of her death and the all-consuming way in which agencies of social control, such as the police, the legal system and medical science collectively determine that the patient's life and death are taken out of the family's hands and become a matter for the experts. Secondly, Kim's death had an impact on both the family and hospital staff. The hospital made every effort to support and assist the family in their grief, but the staff on the ICU were not offered any counselling. This raises the familiar issue of who cares for the carers in situations like this, when hospital staff members are sharing the experiences of the family. Although their experiences are not the same, their need for support may be just

as intense and valid. A member of staff on the unit recalls his
experiences of Kim's time on the unit:

> For the first time in my career, I found myself nursing a
> corpse, but at the same time attempting to reassure family
> members that this was not so. On the rare occasions when
> relatives were not present I felt more stressed, as it seemed
> that to all intents and purposes Kim was dead.

Death in critical care units takes place within a context that is
shaped by a number of forces, both political and social. This reflective incident highlights some of the imponderable issues raised by
a high profile death, which it may be argued was somewhat atypical. It remains the case however that so-called 'high tech' areas
such as A&E departments and renal/heart transplant units are
contexts subjected to different influences when a patient is dying.
In these life-defining contexts, the emphasis is on the maintenance
of life and preservation of the quality of that life at all costs. In
essence this curative ideology influences the way in which nurses
and doctors behave towards the patient, who, as an acute case may
be viewed in a different light to a patient in a different context.

The social management of dying in hospital

Dying in hospital can be socially defined in terms of staff perceptions of the nature of the patient's illness, their attitudes towards
the appropriateness of the impending death and the context in
which terminal care takes place. The time a patient spends dying
and the events involved in the patient's passage from wellness to
illness loosely referred to as the dying trajectory (Glaser & Strauss
1965) also influences the way in which the terminal care is
managed.

When a person is admitted to hospital, a number of factors
influence the way in which he/she is treated, least of all the medical condition and the context in which the treatment takes place.
A wide range of social factors impinge on the way in which a
patient's trajectory through the hospital occurs. The patient's age,
gender, social class, race and ethnicity play a part in shaping the
perceptions of both staff and patients towards the person. Staff

attitudes towards patients with learning disabilities or mental health problems can have an adverse effect on the patient's passage through the hospital. For many patients the process of admission to hospital, especially for the first time, can be traumatic in more ways than one. Goffman (1968) and others have discussed the dehumanising effect of hospital admission which can be very distressing if the patient is not made to feel welcome by the staff. For a number of unfortunate patients their first contact with hospital takes place as a result of an accident or trauma. Admission through A&E departments involves assessment and often facilitates acute treatment taking place, especially if the patient's condition is life threatening.

The following case scenario focuses on age as a social factor influencing a person's experience of hospital. Age is often a key factor in the assessment and initiation of treatment. Similarly, the experiences of some older people in hospital reflect the way in which attitudes about older people can be based on notions about the deserving nature of the patient's condition (Health Advisory Service (HAS) 2000). A young child with rheumatoid arthritis (Still's disease) may be treated differently to the older person with osteo-arthritis. Both conditions are painful and distressing. However, the child's treatment will invariably include acute intervention which may not apply to the older person due to the arthritis being seen as a disease of old age, not susceptible to cure, unlikely to respond well to treatment and may be due to other factors such as obesity, which can be dealt with by the patient themselves. The child's illness may give rise to acute pain and an increase in temperature that can be alleviated with drugs and is likely to resolve with the appropriate treatment. In an adequately resourced health service, both patients would receive treatment and health education to prevent a recurrence, in practice the indications are that age does make a difference in relation to the way that many older people are treated in hospital (Health Advisory Service (HAS) 2000).

Patients entering acute and critical care areas in many cases may be younger than those in other areas, such as elderly care units. Therefore public perception of the 'deserving nature' of their death and the social management of dying may influence hospital staff in considering decisions made about 'end of life issues' particularly if the patient is perceived to have 'had a good innings'.

Age appears to be a significant factor in the management of death and dying along with the patient's gender, race, social class and mental health. In particular for older people perceived to be 'nearer death' their passing may be perceived as 'a blessing' for staff and family alike, depending on circumstances. A frail older person with multiple-pathology and a debilitating stroke may be considered in a different light to the young child rushed into the A&E department. These factors reveal issues not only about the differing context(s) in which dying takes place, but also about the attitudes of hospital staff regarding their own mortality and to a certain extent ageist attitudes towards older people. Evidence from the HAS report (2000) suggests that older people admitted to hospital are often treated in an inferior way to their younger counterparts. The death of an older person in hospital can often reflect the mores of the setting in which death and dying takes place (Costello 2000). The extent to which emergency treatment is initiated depends on the context in which care takes place. Continuing care units often do not have emergency life saving equipment with which to initiate cardiac resuscitation for example, therefore, unlike areas for younger patients with acute illnesses, such life sustaining treatments are not available to older people in certain elderly care contexts.

Summary

This chapter contrasted the reactions of hospital staff to the death of a neonate in maternity where shock and disbelief were blended with profound sadness. When faced with death, the maternity ward context which strives to provide life is challenged to be able to manage effectively the death of a baby which is regarded as a tragedy. The structures, which are normally used to celebrate birth, have to adapt to providing support to the bereaved family and this can be difficult when the overarching ideology is focused on life. The social structures used to help memorialise life such as hand prints and photos of the baby serve as sources of comfort and can enable parents to cope with the crisis. Equally in critical care contexts, where saving lives is the key aim, staff need to be aware that death is ever present. The critical care context can be very constraining when death occurs, as little privacy is available and lay observers are made painfully aware that apparatus designed to monitor bodily functions are everywhere and serve to remind observers of the life saving purpose of ICU. In this critical care context, as the reflective incident of Kim illustrated, staff members can feel constrained from acting individually as there is pressure to work as a team, even though at times nurses and others may feel that the efforts being made to preserve life are futile and the patient should be allowed to die in dignity.

Chapter 2 will examine in more detail the nursing care of dying patients, taking a 'day in the life' approach to the care of terminally ill patients in the hospital context.

Further reading

Clark D. (2000) 'Death in Staithes' in Dickenson D., Johnson M. & Katz J.S. (eds) *Death, dying and bereavement* (2nd edition). Open University Press, Buckingham: 1–3.

This chapter describes the traditional practices that took place at the beginning of the 20th century in a North England town. It is highly regarded as a classic account of the behaviours and attitudes of families at the time of death.

Jupp P. C. & Gittings C. (eds) (1999) *Death in England*: an illustrated history. Manchester University Press, Manchester.

This book includes ten chapters written by different experts and takes a social historical view of death covering a period from the Pre-Bronze age up to and including the death of Princess Diana. The theme of the book is placed on the changing societal attitudes towards death and although very comprehensive and well illustrated is an academic text that chronicles the way in which attitudes towards death reflect changing social values.

Katz J. & S., Sidell M. (1994) *Easeful death*. Hodder & Stoughton, London.

This very readable book is aimed at professional caregivers and covers a wide range of issues relating to terminal care and the management of death in institutional and community settings. The book is easy to read and although it covers a range of topics including communication, symptom control and bereavement support, some are not covered in detail. The authors pose the question what is a good death and challenge the reader to consider some of the practical issues associated with providing effective care to the dying patient.

Seymour J.E. (2001) *Critical moments – death and dying in intensive care*. OU Press, Buckingham.

This is a very interesting and well written book which contains a clear glossary. It is based on the author's doctoral research and professional experience of working in intensive care. The book deals with a number of critical issues such as withdrawing treatment and the notion of good and uncertain deaths. One of the central themes of the book is decision making as a social process and the organisational constraints placed on staff in ICU which serves to support the idea that often individual decisions about patients are rarely made without being influenced by the context in which care takes place.

Walter T. (1990) *Funerals and how to improve them*. Hodder & Stoughton, London.

This is a very interesting, excellent and thought provoking book written in a style that has become popular amongst both academics and lay readers. The book is focused on the modern day funeral and seeks to illuminate on how funerals can meet the needs of a diverse multicultural society. Included in this comprehensive book are chapters on cost, the afterlife and how funerals should be conducted. The author poses basic questions such as what is a funeral?, considers the various ways in which families can adopt a do it yourself approach or deal effectively with what he calls the funeral trade.

Walter T. (1994) *The revival of death*. Routledge, London.

This book is a classic, mainly because it covers topics not considered in such detail before, and also because Walter's writing style has appeal for the academic and lay reader alike. It is extremely well written and fully referenced. The main thrust of the book is placed on highlighting the interest that people have developed in all aspects of death and dying. Walter's argument is based on a reconsideration of the death denying theses and he carefully constructs a case for society not being as afraid of death as it was fifty or so years ago. I highly recommend this book to anyone interested in finding out more about death and dying.

2

Dying in hospital: issues in the institutional care of terminally ill patients

Introduction

Most people in our society prefer to die at home although over 60% of people in the UK die in hospital. Faull & Woof (2002) point out that most hospital resources are used for people in the last year of life and 10–15% of hospital beds at any one time are used for patients with advanced disease with a third of such patients dying within a week of their final admission. Many patients (40%) admitted for terminal care are in hospital for longer than a month (Faull & Woof 2002) and thus it may be argued that much palliative and terminal care takes place in hospital.

This chapter will focus on a description of the care of dying patients in an acute elderly care ward adopting 'a day in the life' approach. The material in the chapter originates from my research study in three different elderly care wards, Cherry, Lilac and Elm where I worked as a participant observer (Costello 2000). By its very nature the care of dying patients takes place within a context that includes the care provided for patients at varying stages of their illness. The 'recovering patients' were often cared for next to dying patients, since nurses in general were reluctant to put dying patients in side rooms and therefore the care of dying patients took place in what may be described as a public environment. By examining the care of dying patients in this way, it is hoped that a number of features of terminal care will be highlighted, such as nursing work and the way in which hospital procedures and ward routines, in themselves, can become more important than the care of patients. This will become one of the major themes of the chapter, the aim of which is to reveal a number of insights into the reality of hospital care for the dying patient. Particular emphasis is placed on the organisation of care in hospital, based on teamwork and how such care becomes problematic when patients are dying.

The chapter looks at the various ways used by nurses to provide high quality care through individualising the provision of that care when a patient's condition becomes terminal. As in the previous chapter, a case study of a dying patient will be highlighted in order to make clear how aspects of nursing care are put into practice and in particular, how the patient's family becomes part of the pattern of care. The chapter will conclude with an examination of the way(s) in which nurses manage the care of the patient after death, by focusing on the nursing procedure known as last offices.

A day in the life of Cherry Ward

Cherry Ward formed part of the elderly care unit of North Hospital, one of the new-wave NHS Trusts with 1100 beds, 180 being dedicated to the care of older people. The unit consisted of eight wards and a day hospital. Cherry Ward was situated on the top floor of an old building that formed part of a decaying, former workhouse. Patients were admitted from home via GP referral, occasionally from the A&E department and often by transfer from one of the other three acute wards. (All the wards in the unit were categorised as rehabilitation, with no continuing care beds.) These three acute wards were situated to the front of the hospital in a new purpose built unit, with the 'old wards' (as they were known locally), situated a few hundred metres away. These acute wards tended to admit more acutely ill patients, who, following initial assessment, were transferred back to the old wards for rehabilitation.

Nursing care on Cherry Ward began in the morning with a ward handover from the night staff to the early shift and ended with the day staff on late duty handing over to the incoming night staff. Invariably nursing work on the ward was organised on a team-nursing basis (Waters 1987). This involved different grades of nurses working together providing care for a group of patients, some of whom were highly dependent and dying and others who were reasonably independent or self caring.

Nursing work on Cherry Ward was allocated between nurses working shifts who were divided into teams, with the early shift having two teams and the late shift one. The night staff consisted of a qualified nurse and an auxiliary, often working separately, but also working together when caring for certain patients, such as those highly dependent. The nursing work on the day shift consisted of meeting patients' physical and psychological needs through the imposition of a variety of routines and procedures which allowed certain activities to take place, such as patients' personal hygiene. Wright (1986:61) points out some of the inherent problems with this approach:

> There is always the danger that patients can be squeezed into fitting in with the routine of the nurses, rather than the nurses trying to adapt their work patterns to their patients' needs.

The routine on Cherry Ward was similar to the other wards and was based on a shift work system. The morning shift was often the busiest time, the afternoons being invariably less active, allowing nurses to spend time with patients, together with the opportunity to catch up with paperwork and administration. The afternoon period was a time when there were more nurses on the ward, where individual and group communication in the form of meetings took place. The early and late shift nurses were also able to complete any outstanding nursing procedures such as wound dressings. After the early shift had left, the smaller number of late shift nurses became involved in the evening meal, and an influx of visitors, that continued up to and including the time when the night shift came on duty.

Invariably nurses during the day attempted to individualise the care they gave to suit the patient, although often because of staff shortages and the high dependency of patients, they were faced with tremendous challenges to ensure that patients' needs were tailored to their particular circumstances. The work pattern may be accurately described as a mosaic that included organisational demands, individual needs and professional ideologies about what constitutes effective nursing care such as the implementation of primary nursing (Wright 1986). An example of some of the tensions that formed part of individual versus organisational needs was the preference of some patients wanting to get up early, insisting to the night staff that they be washed and dressed before the day staff arrive. Others, often not feeling well, preferred to get up later and miss breakfast altogether. In between these extremes, patients' needs were accommodated according to an amalgam of individual resources, ward needs such as medical ward rounds and the individual patient's level of dependency.

The organisation of nursing care in a hospital ward

The hospital study involved working both as an active participant and an observer. This approach worked along a continuum whereby at the initial stages of working on a ward, I adopted an active participant 'roll up the sleeves and get involved' approach. However, after a while it became necessary to adopt a more active observer role, in order to explore what was actually going on around me, and in essence, stepping back from being part of the data itself!

The following descriptions are made from observations of nurses working, as well as from subsequent interviews with staff on all three wards. The observational data were verified, clarified and in some cases negated during interviews with those nurses who had previously been observed.

The observations of nursing work on Cherry and Elm Wards revealed three major areas of nursing work that reflected the way in which nurses worked as a team, as well as having a significant effect on nursing care. First, the organisational design of nurses' work, based on teamwork was not conducive to quality personal care. Secondly, on Elm Ward, the division of labour and the imputed teamwork roles led to heightened tension between team members, with a consequential reduction in the standard of nursing care. Finally, when a patient was regarded as terminally ill, teamwork organisation was not practised; in preference individualised care was adopted. This suspension of everyday practice enabled nurses to become more independent and autonomous in their work role. It was interesting to discover that in relation to nursing work, many of the ward staff believed that they were providing dying patients with quality care when it became more individualised, as Maggie (Staff Nurse on Elm Ward) points out:

> I enjoy working together as a team, but at times it gets me down. I become irritated with having to do work that does not relate to direct patient care, such as when certain

members of staff want the beds made or the trolleys moved out and I want to carry out care for the patients. It causes friction and I know a number of us prefer to do more individual care, I don't care if the beds are not made by lunchtime, as it's more important to meet the patients' needs.

In general nurses on all three wards regarded quality care as personal or individualised, focusing on what the patient wanted and needed at the time. Often, it included carrying out personal nursing care, such as toe nail cutting and hair washing and included spending time with the patient carrying out psychological care and not having to carry out any physical tasks. In response to asking: 'What do you mean by individualised care?' A staff nurse replied:

Individualised care is about getting to know the patient and being able to meet their individual needs, in other words doing what they want you to do for them, like wash their hair and help them with make-up or read the paper, which sometimes you cannot get round to doing because we tend to get stuck doing physical work at the expense of talking to patients and doing more personal care.

As the nurse pointed out, this type of personal care took up a lot of time and was not perceived by some nurse colleagues to be the most effective way to 'get through the work'. The organisation of nursing work on all three wards was based largely around adherence to ward routines. My observations on Cherry and Lilac Wards identified that the routinisation of activity, was an embedded part of the ward culture and an established feature of the customs and practices of the ward, which formed part of nurses' everyday ward life:

I worked in a nursing home before I started nursing and it is very similar, the routine, the washing and dressing, and the only way to get through the work is to have a ward routine.

Although nurses on Lilac Ward identified a number of personal care activities that they wanted to do for and with patients, such as spiritual care, many lacked the confidence or ability to fulfil this role:

> I tend not to discuss things like spirituality with terminal patients as I am a bit out of my depth and I am never sure that's what they want either.

Nurses perceived their inability to discuss patients' feelings and spiritual care issues as problematic, since not all patients were told their terminal diagnosis. Nurses therefore had to exercise caution, when talking to dying patients about their future and tended to avoid any discussion that might cause the patient to question the possibility that they were dying. There was also the problem of patients legitimising the type of relationship, referred to as a therapeutic one, in which nurses and patients raise and discuss issues pertinent to the patient's psychological well-being (May 1992). In order to develop more individualised and therapeutic approaches to care, nurses had to develop ways of circumventing teamwork strategies that were viewed as an impediment to the development of such relationships.

Teamwork and terminal care

Much of the organisation of nursing practice on all three wards was based on teamwork. In particular, teamwork on Cherry and Lilac Wards was effective in meeting organisational goals, but not for giving personalised or total patient care. However, when teamwork was utilised within a framework of primary nursing, comprising sufficient competent nurses to give care, teamwork was seen as an appropriate way of organising that care. The ideal situation for terminal care provision was for individual nurses to care for their own patients:

> I like to have the responsibility for my own patients. This allows me to work out what is best for them according to their individual needs and I can plan my work around them and provide the patient with the type of care that they would hope to get at home.

The adoption of individualised care, allowed high quality terminal care to develop. Nurses on Elm Ward often achieved individualised care, because of the increased staff presence and enhanced skill-mix, although during staff shortages, nurses reverted to collective team-work strategies.

Despite the difficulties experienced by many nurses in striving to give quality terminal care, the observational data illuminates how nurses managed to provide individualised care to dying patients, by suspending teamwork and adopting individualised approaches, in order to give more personalised attention. The sus-pension of teamwork allowed nurses to spend disparate amounts of time with dying patients to temporarily shift their responsibil-ity, from tasks onto people. Nurses on Elm Ward regarded that they delivered good quality terminal care, when they were able to make their own decisions about patient care, as well as having the opportunity of getting to know the patient as a person and devel-oping close relationships with them. Caring for dying patients was considered to be very personal and intimate, especially when the patient was close to death.

'Poorly patients'

On each of the three wards in the study there were patients recognised as being more physically and psychologically dependent than others – for a variety of reasons resulting from their acute medical condition, frailty or because they were dying. These patients, often referred to as 'poorly patients', were considered to be highly dependent on nurses and were often accorded specific attention, with their care and well-being being discussed at length during ward handovers, especially at the end of the day shift where night staff were keen to know details of any poorly patients. In particular when such patients were known to be dying, it was important that their specific terminal care sta-tus was appreciated, both by nurses and doctors. Euphemisms such as 'Tender Loving Care' (TLC) were used to describe the care and in some cases the medical notes documented that cer-tain patients were 'for TLC', often with a number of descriptors indicating that the patient was 'to be kept comfortable'. The following extract from a ward handover typifies the way in which nurses often sought to explain terminal care, particularly those patients who were close to dying – Mary (Staff Nurse Cherry Ward):

> Edna is still hanging on bless 'er. ... We have given her all care and she has had a wash, catheter cleaned, her bottom's a bit red but not broken, she's had mouth care and we gave her a few sips ... she's very poorly but not in any pain, it's a shame really 'cos I think she really wants to go and I think her husband has had enough as well.

The staff nurse's comments indicate that nursing care of this particular patient included physical and psychological aspects, highlighting certain key areas such as skin integrity and mouth care. Reference was also made to the patient's feelings, as well as those of her husband. The care of poorly, dying patients often appeared to focus on physical care, because of the link between pain and distress, if a patient had a pressure sore, this would impact on their overall well-being. Because visiting restrictions were rarely imposed in any way on relatives, it was commonly the case that relatives would visit the patients every day, but much would depend on the relative's state of health and their ability to get to the hospital. Family members and friends therefore, were often well regarded by nurses and their wishes sought on the patient's overall condition and management.

Death and dying on the ward

The observations I made on Cherry Ward were limited to a small number of patients who died, most of whom became very poorly and died following a long period of illness, during which their physical condition deteriorated with death being expected. This type of death, as Glaser & Strauss (1968) point out, is often easier for nurses to cope with. The interview data indicated that most nurses on the ward (eight) also found it easier to cope with dying patients who were not aware of their death, a finding supported by McIntosh (1977) but not others (Glaser & Strauss 1965, Field 1987, Field & Copp 1999). I would contend that age and context are key variables, when considering data on this particular aspect of death and dying. The ward disclosure norms regarding terminal diagnosis, which represent the shared understandings about how much information to give to patients and relatives about terminal conditions, clearly identified that patients were not told their diagnosis unless specifically requested. Relatives were invariably informed when death was expected. Staff attitudes towards death and dying varied, with some atypical responses acknowledging the fact that it would 'Be a blessing for some', to others who lamented on the patient's past life; 'She had a good innings.' Many nurses expressed concern, both about the type of death and the way people died. Keith (Staff Nurse) pointing out that:

> We all expect death to happen, but I find it hard when a patient dies in pain and we can't do anything.

Others expressed a desire for more control over death:

> I can't bear it when people linger and linger it's just so difficult for everyone, relatives and all.

Despite the ward disclosure norms concerning information not being given to patients, most nurses I spoke to felt that patients who were expected to die, knew their diagnosis without being told, a finding others have identified (Buckingham et al 1976, James 1986, Field 1987). When asked about terminal care, many nurses felt keen to control the physical, but said little about the emotional aspects and even less about support for relatives.

The cultural practice on Cherry Ward was to place dying patients in the side room. This was atypical of the other two wards in the study and the rest of the wards on the unit. Their rationale for doing so was more pragmatic than attitudinal, since they also used the side room to isolate infectious cases and if a patient was dying on the ward, they would not transfer the patient to a side room simply because they were dying. The side room was situated opposite the ward office and close to the night nurses station and provided nurses with greater opportunity to observe dying patients at all times. Some nurses on the ward disagreed with isolating patients in side rooms, as they felt it was an attempt to hide death, arguing that dying patients had a right to be nursed on open wards. Dying patients on the other two wards (Lilac and Elm) were invariably cared for on the main ward areas, with side rooms being used for patients with infectious diseases. There was no rigid consensus of opinion however, about the use of side rooms for dying patients. Some nurses preferred to care for dying patients in the side room, because as one staff nurse pointed out:

> It helps everybody really, the family and the nurses who are able to give the care without disturbing anyone and when the patient dies there's less fuss.

It is often difficult to nurse dying patients on open gallery style wards such as Cherry, as it places constraints on both nurses and grieving relatives, who generally want to spend a lot of time at the bedside. The nurses on Cherry Ward used numerous adjectives in their descriptions of terminal care, expressing concern for relief of (physical) pain, limiting suffering and keeping the patient comfortable, the latter being a key feature of their approach to the care of the dying patient. The following case study provides an illustration of the main points emanating from the data.

Reflective incident: the death of Mrs Brown

What follows is a descriptive account of the death of an older female patient (Mrs Brown) who, following a brain stem stroke (CVA), was transferred to the ward from an outlying hospital. The patient had previously been refused admission to North Hospital's ICU because of a bed shortage. Mrs Brown was put on a ventilator in the previous hospital, but taken off on the instructions of both a physician and a neurologist who, following tests, determined that she was brain dead. On the day that Mrs Brown was due to be transferred to Cherry Ward, her daughter (Sandra) was informed that the hospital was going to take her mother off the ventilator and that she would almost certainly die shortly afterwards. Subsequently, this did not happen and Mrs Brown, following extubation, continued to breathe voluntarily and showed no immediate signs of dying.

Mrs Brown was transferred to Cherry Ward and admitted into the side room that had been prepared for her. She was hydrated via an intravenous infusion, with a naso-gastric tube in situ and a urinary catheter on free drainage. She was deeply unconscious, unresponsive to stimuli of any kind and breathing by herself, although her breathing pattern was erratic and noisy. Her eyes were open but not responsive and the overall picture she presented was one of a dying patient. Sandra accompanied her mother and was visibly distressed and very angry. She had been told by the previous hospital that her mother would be dead following the extubation, and she had still not recovered from the initial shock of finding her mother collapsed at home two weeks previously.

Before Mrs Brown arrived on the ward, the staff expressed considerable anxiety about her imminent arrival, on the grounds that they had no biography of the patient and were unhappy about receiving a patient who was likely to be admitted in order to die. One of the major presenting problems was the technological image Mrs Brown presented. Under normal circumstances a patient such as Mrs Brown would be given medication to relieve distress. Physicians in North Hospital did prescribe morphine to patients, even when they had no demonstrable pain. The ward doctor explained that 'It can be used to relieve distress.' Despite the side effect of morphine being to suppress breathing, it was explained that it could also, in some circumstances be used to relax the patient and to stabilise erratic and rapid breathing. The use of morphine in this way could have been seen as a justifiable and sensitive way of sedating the patient, especially for someone who was dying. It was also perceived by the staff to be a reasonable way of dealing with 'terminal restlessness'. Mrs Brown was however not prescribed morphine on her admission to Cherry Ward. As a dying patient, she would also normally have had her naso-gastric tube removed and not been hydrated with an intravenous infusion. In terms of Mrs Brown's presenting image, she did not appear to be dying. The amount of equipment being used to sustain her condition suggested that she was being actively treated.

This contravention of the stereotypical picture of the dying patient presented the nurses on Cherry Ward with a problem, in so far as the patient did not fit their predetermined image of a dying patient. Attempts were made by nurses on the ward to normalise the situation and continue to monitor Mrs Brown's progress, with regular four hourly observations of her temperature, pulse and respiration together with monitoring of her fluid input and output, as the previous hospital had done. Sandra was informed that she could visit anytime and was told by the nurses that her mother's condition would be closely observed. Sandra later admitted to me that she felt very isolated and insecure during the time of her mother's admission to Cherry Ward. She felt that the hospital did little to alleviate her feelings, she commented:

> I got the impression that my mother and I were not supposed to be there.

The nurses on Cherry Ward initially treated Mrs Brown as an unconscious patient, ensuring that all her physical care was given. My perception was that the nurses felt unsure as to how to develop their approach, as she did not seem to fit easily into any known 'patient category'. Nurses on Cherry Ward were used to caring for unconscious patients following a stroke, but these patients had their eyes closed and were often deeply unconscious. One member of staff commented that it was Mrs Brown's appearance that unsettled her. Ann (Auxiliary):

> It's a bit weird really 'cos she seems to be with it in some respects but, she isn't, it's the eyes that put me off.

I observed that nurses spent little time attempting to talk to Mrs Brown (who could not reply) although nurses did report feeling uneasy about her presence on the ward at first. In the ward office at handover time, Mrs Brown became the most talked about patient on the ward. 'Why had she been transferred?' The insensitivity of it, the distress it must have caused her daughter and most of all why were they keeping her alive? Ken, the Junior Houseman was asked about Mrs Brown's treatment. He pointed out that the ward consultant had agreed it was unwise to continue active treatment but was seeking advice from their own neurologist about Mrs Brown's clinical state. However, Sandra saw no reason to continue with any treatment and was becoming increasingly concerned at the confusing picture she witnessed.

When her mother had been on the ward for a week, Sandra began to visit every other day, but would ring the ward daily. Ten days after her admission, the hospital neurologist came to see Mrs Brown, read the notes from the previous hospital and examined her. He agreed that there was evidence of brain death, but stated that he could not confirm categorically that it was brain death until a period of 6 months had elapsed. He advised that Mrs Brown be 'kept comfortable'. Following his visit the intravenous infusion being used to hydrate Mrs Brown was slowed to its minimal input and the nasogastric tube removed. It had been argued by nurses that it affected Mrs Brown's breathing and was not being used for any particular purpose, since the patient was not eating. The night following the visit of the neurologist, the intravenous infusion 'tissued' (came out of the vein); the on-call houseman was reluctant to reinsert it and therefore the infusion was discontinued. The next day the catheter was removed on the basis that it was no longer required. These changes seemed to alter nurses' attitudes towards Mrs Brown: 'She can be treated properly and cared for in a humane way now', stated the night staff nurse at the handover that evening. The night staff expressed relief that Mrs Brown was being treated in what they perceived to be an appropriate way. Mrs Brown continued to be cared for as a terminally ill patient, receiving all physical care for a further 9 days until she died one night in her sleep. Her daughter was relieved, but remained angry about the way the situation had been managed at the previous hospital, stating that she had received misinformation and was insensitively treated.

Care of the dying patient and the family

The nursing care received by many dying patients in hospital, as many authors attest, should include emotional support given to those family members and others who accompany the dying person during their final days of life (Field 1989, Penson 1993, Katz & Sidell 1994). This, however, as Field (1989) points out, is one of, if not the most difficult thing for nurses to do. The death of a family member can and does have a traumatic effect on those left behind, particularly when the family are unable to be at the hospital when the patient died. Young & Cullen (1996:64) describe how one of their respondents felt very comforted by being with the person in hospital, but relieved at leaving:

> I'm very glad to get away from the hospital with patients dying all the time. I was beginning to feel I couldn't think of anything else. In the normal world you don't think about death and dying everyday, but I began to get absorbed by it.

Kellehear (1992) draws attention to the social experiences many families have when one of their members is dying in hospital, as well as the importance of saying farewell. This, he argues, is an under-researched area; calling for a broadening of research, Kellehear maintains that the experiences of families in hospitals tend to be underplayed by professionals, who focus on the specific care given to the dying person.

One of the particular problems I encountered in relation to the previously described case study was that the voice of the family was not heard. Sandra stated that:

> I kept trying to tell them (the doctors) that my mum would prefer to be left alone but they just ignored me.

Clearly, effective terminal care for dying hospital patients takes account of the involvement of families and friends accompanying the dying person. This particular aspect of care provided a challenge for nurses who, as Field & Copp (1999) identify, see interaction with the families of dying patients as a difficult area of their work.

The case study depiction of Mrs Brown highlighted a number of significant issues relating to the death of a patient for whom there was no biography. First the patient's presentation to the ward was atypical. Mrs Brown was transferred to the ward with a history of misinformation and poor management that resulted in a distressed and angry relative, who was feeling deeply shocked and isolated from the social loci of care. Secondly there was ambiguity surrounding the patient's treatment and future medical management. Nursing staff had no control over the patient's admission to the ward or the previous treatment and care received. During the period when the patient was first admitted, it may be argued that she was neither recovering nor terminal. This *'liminal'* (Turner 1967) ambiguous situation appeared to make nurses uncertain about their actions and may account for why they failed to respond effectively to the needs of either the patient or the family. On reflection and with hindsight, if nurses on Cherry Ward had contacted the referring unit, it may be argued that more illuminating details could have been accessed and would have resulted in a joint meeting of nurses and doctors, regarding the specific care of Mrs Brown, but neither of these suggestions were taken up. In the meantime the liminal condition of the patient generated sustained anxiety between the staff and Mrs Brown's daughter. By including the family in a discussion about the care, the nurses could have reduced some of the isolation felt by Sandra. It would appear that Cherry Ward was poorly equipped to deal with patients who present in ambiguous circumstances. Significantly, once the patient's dying trajectory became much clearer, the relief of the staff became almost palpable.

The impact that Mrs Brown's circumstances had on the ward staff, at least initially, may be described symbolically as a pollutant one. She was clearly not a terminal patient, neither was she likely to survive. The lack of assertiveness of nursing staff to seek to relieve the confusion, suggested that medical authority was firmly established on the ward. I could not detect any strong views being made towards the medical staff reviewing the active form of treatment Mrs Brown was receiving. Sandra was clearly unhappy with the active treatment, but felt impotent in getting her view appreciated. At the same time, it may be argued that moral dilemmas such as this create ambiguity about death and cause all those involved to 'freeze' in their cognitive ability to strive for a solution. Perhaps there was no appropriate solution to such a situation. In this patient's case, it was almost as if the imminent death had both a pollutant effect, in that staff seemed to avoid her, as well as there being a desire for her to die soon, in which case the patient may have been seen to have resolved the dilemma for herself.

Mrs Brown's particular situation, although atypical for elderly care wards, highlights a number of issues. First the circumstances in which patients are admitted to hospital and the degree of influence and control nurses have over the type of patients they receive. Secondly, there is a need to consider the communication between agencies, such as other hospitals, in referring patients with complex medical conditions and finally, the death of Mrs Brown highlights the need for hospitals to consider embracing the notion of family care, when presented with patients who are dying in hospital.

Last offices: care of the patient after death

The nursing procedure known as last offices, which takes place after the death of the patient has been a revered activity by many nurses, providing them with a way of expressing their feelings for a patient after death. The nursing care of a patient after death, often referred to as 'laying out' has a long history (Wolf 1988) and has changed considerably since Pearce (1963:120) described the procedural elements:

> As soon as the patient has breathed his last the nurse should gently close his eyes … she should then lead the relatives from the room, and in hospital should then bring sister or the doctor to speak with them.

Cooke (2000) points out that the laying out procedure was based on tradition and ritual and its symbolic significance, as a way of enabling nurses to show their feelings and become involved in the final actions, on behalf of the patient.

In the last decade, last offices as a nursing procedure has been based on ensuring that grooming and the correct identification of the body take place, having less to do with traditional attempts to control infection. In contemporary practice it involves far less intervention by the nurse, placing emphasis instead on the legal issues surrounding death. Traditionally, nurses were required to thoroughly cleanse the body, packing the patient's orifices to avoid leakage of body fluids. Pearce (1963:120) points out that:

> Moist swabs should be provided to cleanse the orifices and wool and forceps if they are to be plugged.

Contemporary hospital practice invariably requires nurses to remove invasive equipment such as intravenous lines, naso-gastric tubes and indwelling urinary catheters, making sure that wounds are covered, so as not to leak.

The last offices I took part in on Elm Ward involved an older man (Dennis) who died following a prolonged bout of pneumonia. After he died we felt it appropriate to leave his body covered for a short period (some nurses felt an hour showed respect, although this time varied according to demand and resources, such as when the shift change was taking place). His wife was with him when he died and after she said her goodbyes and left we ensured that Dennis had his dentures in and washed him thoroughly (despite the fact that the funeral director would do this later). The grooming included hair and nail care as it was important that we made sure that the patient's hair was combed/brushed according to his normal style. Changing the patient's hairstyle can distress relatives who may comment that the person did not look anything like their usual self. One of the aims of last offices, as carried out by Bev (the Auxiliary Nurse), and myself, was to try to get the patient to look as much like their normal self as possible, which can be difficult to achieve at times, due to their medical condition. In the past a paper shroud was used to cover the body, although these days many nurses find these both impersonal and undignified choosing instead to use the patient's clothes such as pyjamas or clothes previously arranged by the patient or the family. Sally (Staff Nurse Elm Ward) remarked:

> I hate using the shroud, as it gives a very unreal impression of the patient and the relatives are often shocked when they see their loved one with a white paper gown on, it looks horrible really, we don't tend to use them at all now, it's much nicer in their own clothes.

There is a bureaucratic aspect to last offices, which involves ensuring that all personal belongings are removed from the patient and accounted for in a valuables book, unless the family have already dealt with these matters. When a patient has died in hospital, those relatives present will invariably say their goodbyes at the time of the patient's death. Others may be contacted by the family and choose to come and say their goodbyes whilst the patient is still on the ward or, in some circumstances, once the patient has been transferred to the mortuary. In these circumstances the procedure known as last offices takes place which involves placing a pillow under the jaw to prevent the jaw gaping open. This can also be achieved by tying a bandage around the patients head and jaw. However, if the pillow or bandage is not removed when relatives come to say their farewells, the appearance of the patient is upsetting and can be very distressing for them. None of the nurses on the wards in the hospital study used the traditional practice of tying the jaw with a bandage around the head, which, although practical, was considered both undignified and unnecessary since a pillow performed a similar function and looked more respectful. Finally before 'wrapping up' the body ready for disposal, the feet are tied together to prevent movement in transit. Traditionally a mortuary sheet was used to cover the patient, with the identification label attached to the outside of the sheet. Many hospital nurses attach wrist bands to the patient and, in my experience, felt pen was used to write details of the patient's name and hospital number on the sole of the foot, so as to ensure identification when the patient was placed in a drawer in the hospital mortuary. Thankfully this practice was short-lived due to the perceived lack of dignity. The common practice in many hospitals is to wrap the body in a hospital sheet and place a name label on the outside of the sheet, prior to collection of the body from the ward.

Nurses on all three wards often pointed out that they saw terminal caregiving as a privilege and many expressed sadness at the death of a patient. Some nurses expressed strong desires to carry out last offices (previously explained), as a final symbolic, respectful practical act. In general, nurses on all three wards saw last offices as a reverent procedure to be carried out quietly, with little talking and with the utmost respect being paid to the patient and their family. This aspect of the procedure may be seen as the common link between the previous and the present approach, towards the care of the patient after death.

Last offices and the care of patients from different cultures

Most hospital nurses are aware of the need to observe certain practices when patients of different faiths die on the ward. Neuberger (1987) makes it clear however that the extent to which a patient may require the nurse to attend to their religious needs depends largely on their beliefs and willingness to adhere to orthodox practices. A common example is the death of Jewish patients in hospital. Some Jewish patients will not wish to have others observe all the cultural practices such as prayers for the dead. Others, more orthodox in their religious views may wish the Rabbi to advise and guide others in enabling the death to reflect their beliefs. When orthodox Jewish patients die on the ward, the Rabbi will invariably become involved before and after the death and will assist nurses in the most appropriate way to observe religious and cultural practices. Many nurses are aware that orthodox Hebrews and some Muslims do not wish Christians or non-Hebrews to handle the body. In such circumstances, the wearing of gloves is acceptable practice should the patient die with no family members present. In these circumstances, some nurses prefer to leave the body until the family arrives, allowing them to determine what they would like the hospital to do. In many cases the family, or their religious advisors, will make the patient's wishes and the cultural practices clear before death.

Death on the ward and disposal of the body

Once the patient is groomed and made ready for transfer to the mortuary, the porters are contacted to come and collect the body. This aspect of death symbolises some of the problems to do with control over the process of dying in hospital. On Cherry Ward when the porters came to collect a patient, the curtains were drawn around the beds and the mortuary trolley was used to transfer the deceased. Once the trolley had gone, the curtains were taken back and 'business as usual' was adopted. At no time did I see nurses discussing what was going on or explaining why the curtains were being drawn. This ritualistic hiding of death took place despite some patients knowing that a death had occurred. It is reasonable to assume that some patients knew what was happening, but chose not to discuss it with the staff, but invariably the patients who knew the patient would collude with the staff in keeping quiet about death. The other two wards adopted a similar pattern of secrecy about the transfer of a patient to the mortuary and would refer to patients who had died as being 'transferred to rose cottage', a euphemism for death.

Saying goodbye and 'viewing' the body after death

An important part of the care of patients who died on the ward was the management of the patient after death. With the exception of those close relatives who were with the patient when they died, relatives may wish to come to the hospital to say their last goodbyes, which were sometimes referred to by hospital staff as 'viewing the body'. The term 'viewing' was mainly used by porters, although it is a term used more commonly by funeral directors when families come to the chapel of rest to 'view the body'. In one hospital, the mortuary consisted of a viewing area into which the relatives are ushered and consists of a glass window through which the relatives look at the patient who is taken from the cold cabinet and placed on a trolley covered with a hospital sheet. The son of a patient who had died on Cherry Ward was unable to get to the hospital for two days because he had been on holiday. Due to staff shortages I escorted the man to the mortuary to view his father. Viewing in the mortuary is not encouraged by hospital staff since, in many hospitals, mortuaries are impersonal areas and not conducive to the expression of feelings. Nurses and porters were often reluctant to become involved in viewing in the mortuary because it was also distressing for family members who in some cases felt guilty for not being there at the time of death. Hospital porters in particular were reluctant to become involved in viewing, since it was often distressing for the family and was an awkward situation for the porter, who did not know the family. Porters often insisted that a nurse be present when viewings took place. Bob (Deputy Head Porter) points out:

> I don't mind doing the viewing after death but some of the lads hate it, it has to be done, but I prefer a nurse to be there, after all we have no training, we don't know the patient and it is a very personal thing to be involved in.

In some hospitals because of staff shortages, it is sometimes not feasible for nurses to escort relatives to the mortuary. The nurses in the study who knew the family would invariably volunteer to go with the family to say their goodbyes, often inviting them back to the ward afterwards for tea and a sympathetic chat and to ensure that they were given the necessary instructions about administration matters.

Summary

Using a 'day in the life' approach, this chapter has described the care of elderly patients in hospital and some of the difficulties of providing and making specific the care of dying patients being cared for in close proximity to recovering patients. The structural processes involved in the provision of terminal care meant that at any time nurses were prepared for death. In other words, nurses used strategies for ensuring death was managed such as disclosing the information to the family, keeping the patient comfortable and ensuring that everyone (except the patient in some cases) knew about the impending death. During ward handovers death was discussed and various codes and rules such as Do Not Resuscitate (DNR) orders were debated. This is invariably a feature of the care of patients in hospital, which nurses find problematic. Simultaneously many patients recover from their illness and were discharged. The structure therefore had to be flexible and enable people to die in dignity. The various nurses involved in care had their own ideas about what may constitute a good death and demonstrated their individual ways of saying goodbye through rituals enacted after the death of the patient. Overall, many nurses struggled to meet the patient's individual needs largely due to problems with lack of staff and resources and the physical and psychological demands of caring for vulnerable patients in a context where individual needs took second place to the demands of the organisation.

In the next chapter a closer examination is made of some of the social processes which underpin the nursing care given to dying patients and involves the relationship between nurse, patient and relatives.

Further reading

Black J. (1991) 'Death and bereavement: the customs of Hindus, Sikhs and Muslims'. *Bereavement Care* (10)1, 6–8.

A very interesting article focusing on the cultural and religious aspects at the end of life. The article outlines the needs of Hindus, Sikhs and Muslims at the end of life and some of the ritual practices observed by families and relatives at the time of death and afterwards during the mourning period.

Cooke H. (2000) *When someone dies: a practical guide to holistic care at the end of life.* Butterworth, Heinemann, Oxford, UK.

This is an excellent and very readable book, which covers a wide range of issues relating to the care of both the patient and the needs of the family at and around the time of death. The book considers the control of symptoms in terminal care situations and the needs of the bereaved. In particular, part four deals with the religious needs of the dying and discusses the care of patients from different faiths and the importance of different religious traditions.

Neuberger J. (1987) *Caring for dying patients of different faiths.* Sainsbury series, Austin Cornish, London.

This book written by a well-known Rabbi sets out to provide information on a wide range of issues relating to people from different religious beliefs. The text covers many aspects of terminal care including spiritual and practical advise on end of life matters both before and after death relating to the dying patient and the family.

3

The hospital as a controlling context

Introduction

This chapter considers the way in which hospital culture influences the way in which doctors and nurses play a role in the social construction of death and dying. Bowman & Thompson (1995:227) argue that organisations such as hospitals 'Have their own culture which may be quite different from the wider society.' One of the key themes of this chapter is that hospital culture, beliefs, values, recurring behaviours and customs impact on the way nurses and doctors behave. When certain parts of the culture are examined such as the organisation of nursing work, it becomes clear from both observational and interview data that it is the hospital staff themselves who play a significant part in the creation and maintenance of the cultural practices of the hospital ward. The chapter takes a critical view of hospital culture as a major controlling influence on the nursing care of dying patients. It reviews not only the way in which hospital rules and values influence behaviour, but also their origins and how nurses and doctors take an active part in the construction of their own culture. In particular, tacit agreements, those unspoken shared understandings between nurses and doctors that help to form institutional patterns of behaviour, and notably the way in which information about death and dying is controlled.

One of the themes of the chapter is the way in which information about terminal diagnosis is given to patients and their relatives. The construction of these 'disclosure norms' for providing dying patients with information, is an example of the way nurses and doctors communicate with patients and their relatives. A number of examples are used to illustrate the way values and beliefs about death and dying are communicated in hospital. By utilising a case study example, the chapter looks closely at how the truth about a patient's terminal diagnosis is concealed. A number of authors have highlighted the relationship between the behaviour of the individual and the organisation and in particular how the latter influences the former. Schou & Hewitson (1998), maintain that interpreting the organisational design, structure and ideology of social institutions (such as hospitals) is an important way of explaining the meaning of awareness contexts. It is important to note that these contexts are perceptions and understandings that people have which help them to make sense of what is going on around them. These authors point out that any sociology of dying must address the issue of how the construction of terminal illness is made and conveyed to the patient. Without such an examination, in a social sense, and likewise for research purposes, the authors argue that the patient would otherwise not be dying.

Dying trajectories

The term dying trajectory was first used in 1965 by American sociologists Glaser & Strauss when they were describing the passage of a dying patient through the various investigations and treatments that constitute medical treatment and nursing care. A patient's death trajectory is a perceived entity and does not have objective reality, although many of the phenomena included in the dying person's trajectory may be based on real events, which Glaser & Strauss (1965) described as *'critical junctures'*. A number of critical junctures can be incorporated into the dying patient's trajectory, which influence the patient's passage towards death. The first of these is the amount of information the person has about their terminal diagnosis; this is a topic debated in more detail in later chapters. The second is the extent to which the patient's illness is likely to be susceptible to medical intervention. The third is whether the patient has control over their hospital treatment and if so, to what degree.

Nurses' perceptions of terminal illness

One of the emerging features of my interview data on the way nurses respond to the death of an individual patient, was the degree to which the death was controlled. Part of the controlling influence, was the notion that the nurse was able to anticipate the patient's death and make preparations for it. This related to notions nurses had about different types of death (Costello 2000). A good death in hospital was one that allowed for a degree of predictability and control where relatives and staff (but not necessarily the patient), were aware of the impending death. Preparations would include providing emotional support for the family and controlling the patient's symptoms, in particular, pain. In the absence of any preparation, death had the potential to disrupt the smooth running of the ward. Central to the nurse anticipating the death of a patient was being able to monitor the patient's progress during the terminal stages and assess the rate of deterioration and relative imminence of death. Nurses on Elm Ward made these judgements with varying degrees of accuracy, but it was impossible to become unequivocal about when a patient would die; such matters were often complex and ambiguous. From an organisational perspective, the accumulation of nurses' knowledge, information and awareness revolved around this type of communication. Nurses appeared to develop their awareness of patients' terminal illness individually and collectively through their own ward communication systems. This evolved from within the structures used to organise nursing work such as team nursing. By providing care to a particular patient over a period of time, nurses when focused on the individual patient, often developed an acute sense of the patient's well-being. Kim (Staff Nurse) pointing out that:

> When a patient is very poorly and dying it can be difficult to know for sure when they are going to die, although it is often easier to pick up if and when they have psychologically 'given up' and it's almost as if they want to die.

Based on ward observations, it seemed as if part of the nurses' evaluation skills focused on an assessment of both the patient's physical condition, such as their vital signs, as well as their intuition based on knowing the patient and becoming aware of their specific needs. One example of this was whether patients who were becoming very ill were judged to benefit from receiving cardiopulmonary resuscitation (CPR) if they had a cardiac arrest. On many occasions, doctors were asked about the resuscitation status of patients who were perceived to be pre-terminal or who were known to be dying. Consideration was given to the effect of CPR on these patients, their chances of survival or whether the intervention would prove futile based on their terminal diagnosis. The decision to initiate CPR often depended on whether the patient was likely to die irrespective of any intervention and whether or not it would be a blessing to 'let the patient go'. This contentious issue featured as part of nurses' perceptions about which patients were regarded as terminal and acted almost as a contingency measure for predicting the nurse's action, should the patient suffer a cardiac arrest. For the medical staff, recognising whether a patient was dying seemed to depend more on an assessment of physical symptoms. Often ward doctors had a clear technical expertise in making decisions about the effectiveness of certain types of intervention and in a medical sense recognising that fatal illness is, as Hinton (1972:58) pointed out:

> Often only too easy, the signs and symptoms may be such
> that a doctor will know straight away that his patient is dying.

Nurses however, because of their close proximity to dying patients, often demonstrate considerable insight into subtle changes in the patient's condition, which often enable them to become aware of when death is imminent. Having knowledge of the patient in this way, may be seen as an important part of the social management of death. Nurses on Elm Ward had fairly clear ideas about those patients whom they perceived were likely to 'do well' in terms of recovering from their illness and those who needed to be closely observed. This ability to know your patients and identify when their condition is deteriorating, was regarded by nurses on Elm Ward as a measure of individual integrity. Being able to make accurate predictions about when they were going to die was much more difficult for both doctors and nurses.

Ward disclosure norms

One of the key issues relating to the care of dying patients concerns the amount of information given to the patient and the family. This has been an area of interest for researchers who have identified that the disclosure of terminal diagnosis plays a pivotal role in the patient's dying trajectory (Glaser & Strauss 1968, Field 1987, May 1993).

The maintenance of ward disclosure norms for informing patients about their terminal diagnosis proved complex and imprecise. Much of what nurses reported to me concerning their perceptions of patients' knowledge of their terminal condition may be constructed from within their conversations with patients. It could also be argued that nurses' perceptions were developed within what Armstrong (1983) has suggested to be, the fabrication of nurse–patient relationships.

With two exceptions, the 41 terminally ill patients in the sample observed during the fieldwork on Elm Ward, were not told their diagnosis by the hospital medical staff. In fact evidence from my interviews with dying patients revealed that many of them 'discovered' that they were terminally ill. The data also suggest that many of these patients did know their diagnosis, but were unwilling to reveal this to the staff on the ward. The attitude of the ward consultant (which formed the basis of the ward disclosure norm), was to tell the patients' relatives both the diagnosis and prognosis. The ward consultant explained to relatives that if the patient asked outright (which only one patient did), then he would tell them the truth about their condition. This ward norm was based on the paternal notion of protecting the patient's best interests. In response to the question posed by the researcher: 'Why are patients not told their diagnosis?' Simon (Houseman) replied:

> Because, in a sense it would cause them to worry and can cause a lot of problems with the family. Obviously in some cases it wouldn't but, if you are going to have a rule, it must be a rule for all, so that, as doctors, we know where we stand.

Simon went on to explain that the norms for disclosure of terminal diagnosis depended on the medical consultant. The establishment of a shared perception on Elm Ward was based around the dominant medical ideology. In this way it may be argued that the establishment of ward norms was part of the socially constructed nature of death and dying in the hospital. The ward consultant determined the disclosure policy on the ward and the rest of the staff, despite having their own beliefs and ideas, largely adhered to it. Many nurses pointed out that most hospital patients find out the truth about their impending death. Ken (Staff Nurse) asserts:

> I am not always happy about not telling the patient they are dying because after a while I think many of them find out for themselves and it makes it harder not to tell them and they often don't want to discuss it with you.

The debate about whether or not to tell patients they are dying is often discussed in terms of patients' rights and nurses' and doctors' moral beliefs. Some believe that we have a legal and moral duty to tell the dying the truth (Hinton 1972). By concealing the truth, the patient may fail to put his/her affairs in order and may unwittingly enter into business relationships that could cause them financial hardship. More importantly there is a need to provide moral guidance and enable the patient to discuss their feelings. These considerations can be matched against the medical beneficence that such knowledge may cause the patient to become depressed or even suicidal, despite there being little evidence to support this view. The consequences of concealing the truth serve to enable nurses and doctors to maintain the (false) belief that the patient (and their condition) is stable and can be controlled.

Withholding information about terminal diagnosis

A consistent feature of the observation data regarding disclosure norms on all three wards was the differing strategies adopted by nurses for withholding information from patients. The interview data suggested that the doctor determined the patient's medical prognosis first, then they (the medical staff), broke the bad news to the relatives. Patients were never told their diagnosis or prognosis directly, although many discovered it for themselves. An exception to this was Mabel who, in advance of having investigations of her liver function, suspected she had cancer and made it clear to her family that 'If it is cancer, I want to be the first to know.' Mabel's family were told the bad news by the ward consultant and then told Mabel. She was unlike most patients, in the sense that once she was told that she was terminally ill, with only several months to live, she refused to stay in hospital. Initially Mabel did not appear unduly distressed by the news that she had cancer and was perceived by the nurses, to be 'in denial'. Mabel made a point of telling anyone who would listen, about her condition, explaining that she had (liver) cancer and was going home to die.

In general terms, taking the lead from the consultant, the nurses did not discuss the true nature of a patient's condition with them, unless the patient specifically asked, which few patients did. A number of patients asserted their suspicions (about their prognosis) with the nurses and myself in ambiguous terms. In response to the question 'Why are you in hospital?' eight patients made the following responses:

(1) 'For tests, all the time tests.'
(2) 'I'm not sure, they think I'm anaemic, I'm not sure it's something else.'
(3) 'God knows. I was unwell feeling "achey" all over and then next thing I'm in here.'
(4) 'Well I'm supposed to have yellow jaundice can you see it?'
(5) 'They say it's a blockage in my bowel but I don't need surgery.'
(6) 'I think it might be some form of tumour of the bowel, they're testing it.'
(7) 'I had a fall but I'm OK, now they're checking my blood pressure.'
(8) 'I have a suspected bleeding in my bowels or so they say.'

Interviews with seven male and one female patient all of whom (I was informed) did not know their diagnosis, made it clear that they knew they were going to die, but chose not to reveal this knowledge to others. Discourse concerning terminal diagnosis was very difficult to develop with patients known to have a terminal condition, but not told by the doctor. In answer to the question 'What is wrong with you?' replies from patients varied, but many indicated that they had some awareness of their condition:

(1) 'I know what's wrong with me an' it's serious but how serious I'm not supposed to know.'
(2) 'I'm dying, well it happens to us all one day but it's no use worrying over it now.'

(3) 'Look, I'm 87 I know what's wrong with me but I put a brave face on, you have to.'
(4) 'It's terminal I'm fairly sure, they won't discuss it but it's clear to me.'
(5) 'I'm very ill, I know I'm ill, it's no good pretending it.'
(6) 'Perhaps I've got a long while to go yet, I don't know, but who does?'
(7) 'It's a cancer, I'm sure of it but are they?'
(8) 'Do I know? well let me tell you, as knows, that it's as clear as day I suspected it long ago.'

The nurses and doctors had a shared perception of what the patient needed to know about their terminal condition. This was based paternalistically on what they felt the patient would understand about their diagnosis. The nurses expressed the view that the disclosure norms were protective in nature. Patients were given information such as: 'The tests were incomplete; there was a bit of a swelling; and the symptoms were due to old age.'

Patients on the ward often developed their own understanding of their medical diagnosis and prognosis. This awareness changed according to the duration of their hospital stay, their experiences in hospital and through interaction with the professional staff. Six patients 'discovered' their terminal diagnosis on Elm Ward over a period of time. These six, although initially unaware of their terminal diagnosis, reported that when 'things stopped happening', such as investigations and observations, they began to suspect that they were not going to recover (suspicion awareness), but chose to keep this information to themselves. It is also clear that many patients have their own lay beliefs about their health problems, which they use to make sense of their medical problems.

The clearest indication that 'something was going on', with patients on Elm Ward was the absence of a discharge date. Discharge planning was an important feature of the organisation of patient care and in its absence it was appropriate that patients who expected to be going home would want to have a date for this. I felt that most of the 39 dying patients (not told their diagnosis by the medical staff) were unaware of their specific terminal diagnosis. Table 3.1 illustrates the researcher's perceptions of patients' level of awareness of their terminal diagnosis.

Table 3.1 Researcher's awareness of patients' terminal diagnosis

Closed awareness	16	(difficult to ascertain in 4 patients)
Suspicion awareness	9	(clear suspicions 'not sure what is going on')
Pretence awareness	10	(7 having become suspicious at some stage)
Open awareness	2	(requested the information then discharged themselves)

(2 patients were unable to make a coherent response to the questions)

The contents of Table 3.1 support the view that the vast majority of patients on Elm Ward were unaware of their terminal diagnosis. This evidence contradicts earlier studies (Field 1989), which suggest that hospital patients in general medical and surgical areas invariably know their terminal diagnosis, although the patient populations in these areas may be considered younger. It also runs counter to the groundswell of opinion, which suggests that in the last decade, a shift has been taking place in relation to adopting a more open discussion of death. It is widely argued that talking about death improves communication and the general welfare of staff and patients (May 1995).

Why conceal the truth from patients?

The interview data derived from the staff on Elm Ward, concerning disclosure of terminal diagnosis, revealed differences in the personal attitudes of nurses about disclosure norms. The majority of nurses seemed ambivalent or indifferent in their attitude to disclosure of terminal diagnosis; at the same time there seemed to be an acceptance by most staff, that patients be 'kept in the dark' about their prognosis. I could not detect any strong feelings concerning consensual agreement about open and/or closed awareness. The data suggested that many of the unqualified staff members had not seriously thought about disclosure as an issue, but student nurses seemed to hold strong views about truth-telling in general and the notion of patient empowerment and advocacy in particular. The most consistent response made by nurses to the question: 'Should competent patients be told their terminal diagnosis?' was 'unsure'. Sylvia commented:

> I really don't know, to me it depends on the individual, I can work it any way at all if they don't want to talk about it, it's fine by me.

One of the significant features of the data analysis was the response made by agency nurses. These particular nurses, who were not part of the permanent staff group (the agency staff) had strong feelings, Anne commented:

> I think people have a right to know their diagnosis whether the relatives think so or not, it is the patient's right to know.

This and other similar views were more reflective of the responses made by the three student nurses on Elm Ward, who felt that patients' rights and empowerment were important regarding knowledge of their diagnosis. It is worthwhile considering that agency nurses were frequently used by the hospital and the elderly care unit in particular. Although they were not employed directly by the hospital, many had experience of working in other elderly care and general medical ward settings. They were also not inducted into the culture and routines of the unit. In this way it may be argued that the ward had its own set of beliefs about sharing information with patients. This was culturally defined within the context of the unit through the shared understandings and culturally induced attitudes of the ward staff. Outsiders, such as agency nurses, may not have shared the attitudes of those who had become familiar with keeping patients 'in the dark' about aspects of their medical treatment.

Overall, the most significant feature arising from the data on nurses' attitudes towards disclosure of terminal diagnosis was the distinct lack of consistency. It appeared from the reported preferences of the ward staff that as a group, they were ambivalent about the maintenance of closed awareness. The medical staff appeared indecisive about becoming involved with dying patients. The ward consultant pointed out that he saw no advantage in medical staff becoming too involved with dying patients; he remarked that:

> I don't know how some of the junior doctors feel sometimes, when it comes to dealing with a dying patient. Personally, I feel as if they look to me for more guidance when it's them who often deal with death on a day-to-day basis. It's something they are not good at to begin with.

In practice, few patients were told their diagnosis, and if they were, it was made clear by the consultant that it was not the nurses' responsibility to tell the patient the truth about their condition. Medical staff on the ward generally adopted a 'this is what is done here' approach to the disclosure of terminal diagnosis, which seemed to emanate from the ward consultant.

Case study: David

David, a 72 year old retired Surveyor is the central character of this case study. He was admitted to Elm Ward with a history of chronic respiratory illness, having been an in-patient on other wards in the past. On this occasion he was admitted with cirrhosis of the liver, a chronic condition involving enlargement, damage and scarring of the liver and an inability to remove toxins from the body, resulting in a swelling of the abdomen (ascites). His condition was treatable, but had deteriorated due to continued alcohol abuse, poor nutrition and dehydration, as he had become unable to make any meals for himself.

The aim, in describing this scenario, is twofold. First it reveals the unfolding of awareness contexts, between an older dying patient and the nurses of Elm Ward, through a description of the case study component and secondly, it allows for an explanation and elaboration of the data, by examining events which took place. The people most involved with David were: Celia his daughter; Sid, his nephew; and Angela, his Primary Nurse. David's wife had died 6 years earlier, having cared for David ever-increasingly in the previous 10 years. Relationships between David and Celia were amicable, despite being unhappy about her father's drinking and the effects this previously had on her mother, who was forced to look after him. Since his wife's death David's drinking increased at the expense of an adequate diet. The provision of meals on wheels did little to improve his diet, as he invariably refused to eat them or to answer the door. Recently, according to his daughter, he had been drinking approximately half a bottle of whisky a day, which he claimed was 'moderate' and medicinal.

Angela (Staff Nurse) admitted David to the ward and informed him that he would undergo medical investigations, designed to measure the extent of his liver failure. Having achieved this, the treatment plan would be to provide him with a good diet, supplemented by a course of vitamins. In conjunction with abstention from alcohol, it was hoped that this would enable his liver to 'have a rest' and begin functioning sufficiently for him to be returned home, in a few weeks' time. David was a difficult patient to develop a rapport with and many of the staff found him difficult to handle. At his worst he could be belligerent, rude and un-cooperative, at his best he was shy and reserved. The strategy I observed being adopted by the staff for handling David was to avoid him as much as possible. Angela, commented that:

> I don't dislike him, it's just that sometimes you just can't seem to get close to him, and it's their choice, so I just play it by ear.

David was placed in the first bay on the ward in a central position where he could be observed. Everyone entering the ward had to pass his bed, but few interacted with him. This seemed to support the view that David was an unpopular patient. His daughter and nephew visited regularly and at no time during the initial 5 weeks, were they given any indication that David was terminally ill.

Closed awareness
At no point was it made clear to David that his condition was treatable, equally it was never made clear that he would not be treated. One of David's physical problems was the build up of fluid in his abdomen (ascites). This was treated symptomatically by drawing off fluid under local anaesthetic, using a needle inserted into the abdomen (known both as a paracentesis and a tap). This did not cure the problem, but acted in a palliative way to ease his discomfort. David had this procedure carried out several times during his stay, but each time he did not ask questions about his condition. The uncertainty of his predicament meant that the physicians were able to prevaricate about what to do with him. Even though David's physical condition could be measured in terms of biochemical analysis, there was growing uncertainty about what to do regarding the impending threat to his mortality. Neither doctors nor nurses really knew what was going to happen to David. The nurses were sure that he was unlikely to be cured, but were uncertain about how long he would live and what quality of life he might have. David was 'kept in the dark' about the fact that he was terminally ill. In a similar way Sudnow (1970:206) found evidence that doctors, treating patients whose

medical conditions bordered on being terminal, were reluctant to discuss the prognosis, as it may reflect their own failure.

After his initial admission to the ward and before his condition deteriorated, David was, as Turner (1967) identified '*betwixt and between*' neither a recovering nor a dying patient. This 'liminal condition' influenced the way in which others came to regard his final status passage to death. David's condition deteriorated and he became more belligerent towards the staff that made efforts to avoid him as much as they could. The fluid in his abdomen continued to accumulate and he became more uncomfortable, refusing to conform to his nursing regime, unless particular nurses, whom he liked, were present. One morning during the ward consultant's round, Adam, the Medical Registrar reluctantly agreed to carry out a further paracentesis, as a palliative measure. The proviso being, that he would only do it if, by the end of the week, David's condition had not improved. Adam's reluctance was related to the growing pessimism shown by the medical staff, who felt that David was a 'hopeless case'. At this stage I was told that the medical staff were convinced that David was dying. I asked Steve, the Houseman about David and he told me that whilst it was not general knowledge about his condition, he considered David to have only a few weeks left to live. David was very unlikely to leave the hospital unless he decided to die at home. The closed awareness pattern was confined to the nurses, doctors and Paramedical staff (PAMs), who treated David daily for a chest condition. David appeared to be ambivalent about his illness. He was more concerned with surviving on a day to day basis. Like many hospital patients, these self perceptions David made about his illness were based upon the experiences of other patients and their perceived condition, which were used as benchmarks in order to self assess his condition. In response to the researcher's question: 'How are you feeling David?' David replied:

> Oh you know, much the same can't complain 'cos if you do nobody takes much bloody notice in this place; at least I'm not as bad as the old chap over there, they had to call the doctor last night, he was in such a bad way.

This comment by David and others made by older patients on Elm Ward, relating to the way patients make sense of their condition, suggested that patients used the physical condition of other patients to make sense of their own illness. Institutional settings such as hospitals where patients die contain both recovering and dying patients being cared for together, such as those on Elm Ward. This could cause the parameters between illness and recovery to become blurred. Further, patients construct their own sense of reality from their environment. The use of closed awareness as a disclosure norm, kept patients like David, 'in the dark' about their condition.

'Blocking out' the dying patient

At the end of the week the results from David's blood test revealed no significant change in his liver function. Adam, the Ward Registrar decided not to carry out a further paracentesis on David, because he was afraid of the consequences, namely that he might die during the procedure. At the ward round the following Monday, the ward consultant partly explained this to David, by telling him that he might be made more uncomfortable as a result of the procedure. David protested that he couldn't possibly be in any more discomfort. The consultant told David that he would prescribe more painkillers and review the situation at the end of the week. David's morphine was increased, he was not convinced that all was well and felt that he was being fobbed off:

> Why won't they do it and get it over with? It's not as if it will kill me to have it done, I've felt worse in my time.

Over the next week the nurses increased their avoidance tactics; observations of his pulse, blood pressure and temperature were either not taken, or taken intermittently. Medical staff remained vague and non-committal towards David, this was in part due to the natural tendencies of the hospital staff to hide and maintain the hidden truth from patients. Everything could be made plausible; '... awaiting test results', became one of the catchphrases used to explain the delay in decision making. It appeared to me that David was less than happy with the explanations he was being given about his condition and was becoming suspicious about what was really wrong with him. 'Suspicion awareness' as Glaser & Strauss (1965:147) have described, is very difficult to maintain and is an unstable situation:

> The dangers of disclosure are very great unless the patient dies quickly or becomes permanently comatosed.

The structural conditions around which David's closed awareness had been maintained began to disappear. Instead of being reassured by the words of the doctors and nurses, David began to question their validity and distrust their accuracy. Nurses new to the ward were told at the ward handover that David was not aware of his condition and it was made quite clear to them that he was not to be told. The lack of intervention by the medical staff and the supplementary tactics of avoidance used by nurses, such as controlling non-verbal gestures and blunting any kind of emotional expression during their interaction with David, served to reinforce the observer's view that something was being kept from him:

> David, to Sue (Staff Nurse): I'm not getting any better am I?
> Sue: Oh what makes you say that, I think you look better than you did yesterday.

The nursing staff on day duty seemed clear that when all the test results were examined, the doctors would do something to improve David's condition. The night staff, who had as much involvement with David as the day staff, because of his position by the night staff's desk, gave him the impression that it was perhaps better not to have a paracentesis carried out because of the risks. David's response to this was:

> But what if they decide not to do the tap at all, then where will I be?

The effects of the increased morphine dose had reduced his discomfort and this at least, helped David's daughter tolerate her father's increasing agitation. David appeared to become more passive as the morphine relieved the discomfort, at least during the daytime. The night staff had requested a further increase in morphine, as David often complained of being in pain at night.

At the next ward round, it was decided that David was well enough to have a further tap carried out, which Adam (the Registrar) carried out. A litre of fluid was removed from David's abdominal cavity, much to the relief of everyone concerned. The procedure was very uncomfortable for David who was exhausted afterwards, but having been given additional morphine, slept well that night and awoke in the morning drowsy and dulled by sleep and drugs. David refused to have a wash, preferring instead to be shaved and change his pyjamas. He expressed relief at having survived the paracentesis:

> Not that anything has changed … I don't think they will do it again, but at least I know the score now.

This last reference suggested that David had drawn some conclusion about his condition from the events of the last 24-hours. In response to the researcher's question 'What do you mean you know the score?' David responded 'Well, I don't think they really wanted to do it at all … What's the point it's only going to happen all over again.' This despondent note reflected his current feelings of having just been through a difficult ordeal, together with the influence of morphine. The rest of his day passed quietly with his daughter and nephew visiting in the evening, relieved to see him more peaceful having survived the ordeal of the paracentesis. Adam explained to David's daughter during visiting, that the tap had been a palliative measure designed to make David feel better, but emphasised that it would not change anything.

The night staff found David pulseless and not breathing; the houseman on call pronounced him dead early the next morning. The cause of death was recorded as myocardial infarction (heart attack), secondary to cirrhosis of the liver and Chronic Obstructive Airways Disease (COAD), a chronic respiratory disease. His daughter refused permission to have a post-mortem carried out, despite a request made by the ward consultant, who came to the ward to speak to her. He explained that David's death was not unexpected and that despite being reluctant to carry out the paracentesis earlier he felt that in the end, it had been the right thing to do for her father and he offered his sympathies. Celia acknowledged the efforts made by the staff and thanked them for caring for him so well, adding that he was a difficult man to look after.

Reflections on David's death

The events leading up to David's death caused the patient and the family considerable anxiety, far more than I can articulate here. The maintenance of closed awareness caused sustained uncertainty for his family, who realised that if David had asked the doctors outright what was wrong with him, they would have told him. The ambiguity about present and future treatment caused considerable anxiety amongst those involved with his care, in particular David. Elm Ward and its disclosure practices directly influenced the feelings of the family and added to the distress of the patient. Telling the family the prognosis and not the patient, caused communication problems between the patient, his family and the ward staff. David's case study reveals that the interactions of doctors and nurses play a significant part in shaping the experience of dying. The anguish, the uncertainty and the 'blocking out' of the patient, can be seen as part of the overall socially constructed experience of dying which this chapter has attempted to describe. This type of social construction between the family and the professionals involves collusion between both groups. At the same time, the patient's awareness of what is wrong with them (in David's case his changing perception from closed awareness to suspicion awareness) adds to the poor communication between hospital staff and patients. The outcome can often result in a lack of confidence and trust between the patient and the staff and, in some cases, the patient's relatives. Based upon my conversations with David, it seems as if David knew he was going to die, but chose not to discuss it openly with his family or the ward staff. The collusion between David's family and the hospital staff (it may be argued) could have played a significant part in David's lack of knowledge about his condition (closed awareness). This absence of the truth caused David anxiety and distress partly due to the perceived lack of information and also because of the prevarication about his treatment. The case study reveals that closed awareness developed into suspicion awareness, which in turn, resulted in a period of sustained uncertainty. This was at the time medical staff were unsure about whether to carry out the paracentesis or not. My experience of David's time in hospital leads me to believe that towards the end of his life, he chose not to reveal what he knew about his terminal diagnosis to his family or the medical staff (pretence awareness). This seemed to be his way of dealing with the realisation that he was going to die, especially when the professional staff in the hospital created no opportunity for him to openly discuss his feelings.

Summary

The chapter highlighted the psychosocial needs of dying patients and the cultural norms used by doctors and nurses to control information. The construction of disclosure norms is a good example of the way structure is shaped by those with the power. Nurses and doctors as agents of social control make decisions about patients, often wishing to act in the patient's best interests. But what are the patients best interests? Communication about death and dying has always been a sensitive issue for nurses and doctors. In the case of David, it may be argued that he was able to make his own decisions but the disclosure norms of the ward prevented this and had a constraining effect on allowing him to decide about his future. The structuring of patterns of care such as disclosure criteria is an example of the way institutional norms can disempower patients and in some cases individual staff members.

Further reading

Field D. & Copp G. (1999) 'Communication and awareness about dying in the 1990s'. *Palliative Medicine* 13(6), 459–68.

This interesting article examines the way in which information about dying is communicated in hospital and 'revisits' the work of Glaser & Strauss (1965), updating and reviewing its validity in relation to modern palliative care. The authors develop the early work of Glaser & Strauss adding another dimension (conditional awareness) to the original work based on their own extensive research in this area.

Glaser B.G. & Strauss A.L. (1965) *Awareness of dying*. Aldine Publishing, Chicago.

This book is a 20th century classic describing the authors' now famous theory of awareness contexts derived from fieldwork research in three San Francisco Hospitals in the early 1960s. The book describes four awareness contexts in which dying can occur. These contexts are theoretically derived from the research, but over time, this conceptual framework has enabled sociologists in general and researchers around the world to make sense of some of the communication problems arising from end of life issues.

Seale C. (1999) 'Awareness of method: re-reading Glaser & Strauss'. *Mortality* 4(2), 195–202.

This thought provoking article sensitively reconsiders the importance of Glaser & Strauss's work and critically reviews the original work considering Glaser & Strauss as '*technicians of interaction*' who prescribe a set of ideas about how to die well in hospital. The article is lively, stimulating and thought provoking.

Timmermans S. (1994) 'Dying of awareness: the theory of awareness context revisited'. *Sociology of Health and Illness* 16(3), 332–39.

This article reflects back on the Glaser & Strauss framework questioning and developing the original work in the light of the authors' personal experience of loss, illuminating some of the more obscure areas of Glaser & Strauss's work and challenging some of the assumptions made in their original research. The balance between personal anecdotal data and insightful observation of the literature makes the article an important contribution to the debate on communication and awareness at the end of life.

Part II
Caring in a hospice context

Part II describes hospice care and consists of Chapters 4 and 5. Both chapters are based on evidence from the participant observation study carried out during a 4 month period in the spring of 2001 at the Beeches (a 12-bedded hospice) (Costello & Horne 2003). Chapters 4 and 5 are focused on the outcomes from the study, which examined nursing work in a hospice context. In broad terms Chapter 4 is more descriptive and adopts a comparative approach. This is not intended as a strict comparative analysis since the hospital and hospice contexts vary tremendously as each chapter demonstrates. Chapter 4 focuses on the palliative care approach from a hospice context and includes a brief look at the origins and philosophy of the hospice movement. The main thrust of the chapter takes a 'day in the life' approach to the nursing management of patients in the hospice. This provides the reader with an overview of the main features of hospice care including the perspectives of patients, relatives and hospice staff and is complemented by an account of a patient admitted for respite care.

Chapter 5 looks at some of the theoretical issues that impinge on the provision of hospice care. Within this chapter, a critical review is made of the contribution of the hospice movement in relation to the management of death and dying. In particular, using case study scenarios, the chapter considers contrasting views of what is referred to as a good and bad death within the hospital and hospice contexts. This chapter attempts to answer the question of why after nearly thirty years of hospice care, does hospital care not match the high standards found in hospice settings? This chapter also examines the issues surrounding the idea of attempting to import hospice philosophy and ideals into hospital settings, especially when considering the work of hospice palliative care teams and the problems associated with the ever changing hospital culture. In broad terms, Chapter 5 is more analytical and reflects on the nursing care provided in the hospice, examining in particular the psychological care, posing the question of whether the principles upon which hospice ideology is based, could ever be incorporated into hospital care?

4 Death and dying in a hospice context

Introduction

Hospice care in the UK is held up as a model of excellence throughout the world and the expansion of what has become known as the hospice movement has made significant advances in the care of dying patients. Despite this, Ellershaw & Murphy (2003) point out that only 12% of patients in the UK die in a hospice. This chapter provides the reader with an overview and insight into the provision of nursing care in a hospice context. It does this by describing the organisation and nursing care at the Beeches, a modern 12-bedded in-patient and day hospice facility. Hospice care will be described, and the origins of the hospice movement outlined.

A 'day in the life' approach sets out to provide the reader with a clear view of hospice nursing. Differences and similarities in care are highlighted and the reader is made aware that in many ways hospital and hospice care are almost incomparable. However, throughout the chapter, I highlight where some of the major differences occur, for example the enhanced resources available to hospices and how this influences the provision of care, such as the pace of work, and the extent to which the environment can and does improve the quality of care. This chapter also reviews staff morale and teamwork structures by considering the way in which patient workload challenges nurses and doctors to work as a team. Multi-disciplinary teamwork is a well-known feature of palliative care in general and hospice care in particular, but is perhaps more difficult to introduce into hospital contexts. The chapter also provides the reader with a patient's perspective, in the form of an authentic case study based on a typical patient (an older man admitted for a short period of respite care), in order to highlight staff responses.

The origins of the hospice movement

The popular conception for many people is that hospices were established in the 1960s as a result of the neglect of dying patients in hospital. However, hospices for dying people were being established in the 19th century when many of our district general hospitals were being built, an example of this being St Joseph's Hospice in Hackney. The financing of such initiatives largely came from public subscription. Ahmedzai (1993) points out what he views to be the second phase of hospice building, which commenced with the opening of St Christopher's and coincided with a time when people were beginning to see flaws in the British NHS. Historically it may be argued that the hospice movement developed out of dissatisfaction with a health care system that was unable to achieve good standards of pain and symptom control (Clark 1993, Walter 1994).

The modern hospice movement originated from the work of a small number of medical professionals disillusioned by the bureaucratic NHS that was unable to communicate effectively with those it served (Lawton 2000). Despite their ability to provide high standards of terminal care, hospices have developed a 'halo effect' whereby others, particularly recipients of hospice care, see health professionals such as nurses, as angels who do wonderful work. As a result of my experiences of volunteer work at St Christopher's, I have learnt that hospice care can produce its own problems, as one staff nurse pointed out:

> It's alright being seen as wonderful but everybody expects you to be wonderful all the time and produce wonderful results which sometimes we don't.

Within this chapter there are several instances where nurses discuss a range of difficult challenges and frustrations they face whilst attempting to control some of the patients' symptoms, as well as the inherent problems shared by NHS colleagues when the hospice is short staffed. Clark (1993:172) points out that the providers of hospice care have developed a reputation for excellence which he refers to as the 'halo effect' of hospice care:

> It is perhaps unforgivable to speak critically about those who make a particular commitment to care for dying people.

The Beeches

The Beeches was opened in 1999 as a 12-bedded purpose built independent hospice together with a day hospice facility for 15 out-patients. The internal layout of the hospice consists of eight single rooms looking out onto a small man-made lake, together with two double rooms. All rooms have en-suite shower and toilet facilities. There were 24 nursing staff led by a full time matron at the hospice, together with a part-time medical director supported by a team of six general practitioners, who work varying shifts in order to provide 24-hour medical cover. Nurses worked an internal rotation shift system between day and night duties. The nursing organisation consisted of staff deployed in two teams (Blue and Green). Each team consisted of a qualified nurse leading a number of Health-Care Support Workers (HSWs).

The medical director herself was a down to earth person who felt strongly that modern medicine had '*lost its way*'. She pointed out that:

> As a healing art medicine today as practiced in hospital, reduces doctors to technicians whose role is to get people out as quickly as possible and leaves very little margin for compassion and proper diagnosis.

The medical staff I spoke to are aware of the diversity of their roles and acknowledge the nature of hospice work, one doctor pointed out that:

> When I worked in the hospital I was inclined to be fast at my work and even a bit aggressive and I suppose in my general practice I am different to the way I am when I come here. I sense that at the hospice people do not expect miracles, but support and good symptom management which is what we do best.

The medical staff at the hospice appeared to enjoy their work and the opportunity it provided them to practice what one called '*human medicine*'.

Patients were referred to the hospice by GPs, district nurses and Macmillan nurses, as well as by hospital medical staff and the hospice day unit. There is invariably respite care provision for at least one or two patients, the admission criteria allows for a 2-week stay unless during this time the patient's condition deteriorates, in which case they stay longer, often until they die. The majority of patients have a cancer diagnosis although patients with non-cancer conditions, such as Multiple Sclerosis are also admitted. To date, no HIV positive patients have been admitted to the Beeches. During the 3-month period of the hospice study the in-patient unit had a total of 89 admissions (see Table 4.1).

Table 4.1 The Beeches: admissions and discharges (day care and in-patient unit) 1 January–31 March 2001

Admitted to day care	16
Discharged from day care	3
Admitted to in-patient unit	89
Discharged from in-patient unit	37
Numbers of deaths	52

Average age of patients admitted to the in-patient unit was 69, with the youngest being 37 and the oldest 93.

The organisation and provision of nursing care at the Beeches was encapsulated within the hospice mission statement (Figure 4.1) which sets out the philosophy and ideology of the hospice. This was based upon Saunders' (1988) concept of '*living until you die*' and although reflecting the beliefs of all the staff, was largely the creation of the hospice matron. The matron's role at the Beeches was multiplex and consisted of taking managerial responsibility for both the day hospice and in-patient units. I did not see the matron become involved directly in clinical nursing, although when patient dependency increased, she adopted her clinical role. The matron's role at the Beeches involved regular liaison with other members of the hospice administration, including the fund raising and hospice executive committees. This called for both diplomacy and integrity. Most, but not all modern hospices have matrons, although many allocate aspects of the role to a range of key members of hospice staff.

A hospice is not just a building but a whole philosophy incorporating care, love and understanding for patients and their carers.
We aim to offer understanding and support – which enables the patients to achieve the best quality of life, appropriate to their individual needs and wishes, throughout the changing phases of their illness, responding and acknowledging to the particular needs of their families and carers by providing high quality care, ensuring comfort and personal dignity at all times, whilst their needs and those of their carers, are met with friendship and understanding.

Figure 4.1   The Beeches mission statement

The organisation of hospice care

The Beeches employed 24 nursing staff on both the day hospice and in-patient units, with half of these being qualified nurses comprising the following grades: one (acting) G; two Fs; five Es, four D grades and seven HSWs. The day hospice had one F grade sister, one E grade staff nurse and three HSWs. All the staff on the in-patient unit undertook internal rotation to night duty with the exception of one staff nurse and one support worker who worked exclusively on night duty. Qualified staff worked closely with and had responsibility for HSWs with the role of the HSW closely resembling that of a nursing auxiliary working in hospital. Most of the HSWs had previous hospital experience with one exception and all had undergone basic induction training. As a group they also received clinical supervision. Volunteers were an integral part of the hospice and undertook a range of duties, including day hospice voluntary work, administration and generally supporting the nurses at the Beeches to a large extent. On most days, the in-patient unit had a volunteer who acted in much the same way as a hospital ward clerk, by assisting and providing administrative support to the nursing staff.

The hospice itself was small and compact with the ground floor kitchen and dining room closely situated to the in-patient unit administrative areas. There were always relatives and friends in the hospice, either because they were accommodated in the living area or were visiting for a prolonged period. This gave the impression of informality with visitors frequently coming and going throughout the day.

The nurses' station was central and within easy reach of the rooms, each of which was equipped with a nurse call button that patients and visitors were encouraged to use in order to summon nursing assistance. The nursing station was located in front of the office, that held the medical notes and functioned as the room where handover meetings at the end of each shift took place. The remainder of the facilities included a multi-faith room, which resembled a small church that had an altar and crucifix at the front, together with a copy of the Bible, the Holy Qur'an and the Bhagavadgita. The multi-faith room also housed copies of the hospice book of remembrance and book of memories. These books identified in the written form, those who had died since the hospice opened in 1999.

Day hospice

The day hospice was open to 15 patients and their families 4 days each week. Referrals being made by GPs, Macmillan nurses, district nurses and in some cases by patients themselves. The latter were asked to contact their GP, who then verified their medical condition before admission. The aim of the day hospice was to provide symptom control and psychological support to both the patient and the family through a holistic assessment process. Typically patients arrived at the day hospice at about 10.00 hours, stayed for lunch and left by 15.00 hours.

One of the common misconceptions about day hospices is that they function in a similar way to the more well-known day hospitals. The day hospital concept is an integral feature of most hospital trusts and tends to specifically cater for older people, providing this client group with social therapy. Modern-day hospices however, focus on the provision of palliative care symptom control, assessment and psychological support for patients and their families. Social therapy, in terms of recreational activities such as painting and pottery served as diversional activities for patients and were considered by the staff to be only a small part of the service provided. The Beeches day hospice consisted of a multi-disciplinary team of seven part-time staff including a social worker, a physiotherapist and her assistant, and four nurses led by Jane an F grade sister; who as the only staff member working 4 days, often coordinated the role of others, as well as playing a significant role in supervising other staff members. Jane was keen to point out that:

> Patients attending the day hospice are assessed according to their needs and are provided with opportunities to see a member of medical staff, a social worker or physiotherapist, our emphasis is on psychological support for those experiencing the cancer journey.

The care provided at the day hospice which had 60 patients, was based on holistic assessment and was not just the road to terminal care. Some of the patients attending the day hospice also received palliative care treatment, such as chemotherapy or radiotherapy and attended the day hospice for assessment and monitoring. The day hospice provided a range of treatments including wound management, blood tests, lymphoedema management and care of central venous lines (for patients receiving cancer treatments). The day hospice staff were also trained to provide sensitive listening skills both to patients and their relatives. Patients were able to see medical staff, as well as the physiotherapist for treatments such as hydrotherapy. Other complementary therapists provided reflexology as well as a range of other therapies, including acupuncture. These therapies were provided on the basis of assessment, in order to meet the therapeutic needs of the patient to enable them to gain effective symptom relief. Patients and family members were also able to seek expert advice from the social worker based in the day hospice who provided information on allowances and other financial assistance for patients receiving hospital treatment. The hospice also provided transport for patients attending the day hospice.

Many patients came to the day hospice for both advice and support but also to meet other patients in an environment of social recreation. The hospice social worker was available for all patients at the Beeches and was based in the day hospice. Together with other staff members, the social worker was the coordinator of a bereavement support group that met on the first Friday of each month in the day hospice lounge. This group offered support to bereaved family members in an atmosphere which fostered listening and encouraged the sharing of feelings/experiences with others who have either undergone, or were still undergoing grief.

One of the newer initiatives being developed by the day hospice was the formation of the '*branching out club*', which was a 'drop-in' facility open for 2 hours each month focused on existing or ex in-patients, together with those considering attending the day hospice. The function of the club was to develop a social forum for exchanging ideas and sharing views amongst patients and family members.

A day in the life of a hospice

The early shift at the Beeches commenced at 07.15 hours with nurses arriving to receive the morning handover from the night staff. All handovers took place in the office, with one nurse 'keeping an ear out' for patient call bells. The night staff discussed those patients who required attention during their shift and discussed the general progress of all the patients. The internal rotation system between all shifts enabled nurses to have insight into the care given to patients during both shifts. Should a patient die during the night it could create a lot of work and activity in the hospice. Staff Nurse Hannah pointed out:

> At night it is usually fairly quiet as we try to keep it like that but if a patient dies we can be busy for several hours with both the patient, the family and other relatives including chaplains. It can be very stressful especially if you do not really know the family that well.

Unlike my experiences of hospital care, I did not encounter any friction between day and night staff. This was largely due to the fact that there was no discernible difference between the two groups due to internal rotation. I did not come across an 'us and them' situation unlike in my hospital research where the day staff often blamed the permanent night staff for problems they encountered, after the night staff had gone home and vice versa (Costello

2000). In general, staff at the Beeches were very supportive of each other, but I also recognised that they were unlikely to express their disquiet about other staff members to a person who may be regarded as an outsider.

The morning shift

After the handover, nurses discussed and planned their work for the morning based on patients' needs and staff availability. The concept of '*the patient day*', referred to by some writers (Wright 1986) as a series of routines based on organisational needs, was not an explicit part of the care at the Beeches. Unlike hospital ward routines, which were structured to take account of medical consultants ward rounds, out-patient appointments and surgical lists; nursing activity at the Beeches was unencumbered by such interventions, although meal times and hospital appointments were an integral feature of some patients' stay. The nursing work at the Beeches was however much more patient centred than I had encountered elsewhere.

In a similar way to many other health care settings, nurses at the hospice were often busier in the morning than the afternoon, in terms of the amount of clinical patient activity. This was reflected in the number of staff on an early shift (five) and on the late shift (three–four). These levels fluctuated according to a range of factors such as staff sickness-absence and in particular patient dependency. During periods of high patient dependency the matron adopted a more clinical role and staff were asked to work extra shifts, such as long days in an attempt to cover shortfalls. This, in my experience is not unusual in a number of hospital settings, such as high dependency, intensive care and operating theatres. However, elderly care settings lack this degree of flexibility and nurses were often left to carry on despite inadequate staffing levels during periods of excessive staff sickness-absence.

One of the more noticeable features of nursing work at the Beeches was the lack of urgency in ensuring that patients were up and dressed in the morning. The earlier part of the morning between 07.45 and 09.00 hours consisted of giving out breakfast to those patients awake but not necessarily up and about. Another striking feature was the quiet atmosphere, unlike many hospital wards where nurses rhetorically pointed out to me that patients had a choice of when to get up, but in practice my observations indicated that there was so much noise going on that it was unlikely that any patient would be able to sleep! The noise of a busy hospital ward was due to the number of patients, their diverse medical treatments and a range of hospital personnel, including occupational and physiotherapists, phlebotomists and medical staff, all of whom were eager to gain access to the patient.

Many patients at the Beeches had breakfast in bed, or at the bedside in their room. Breakfast consisted of cereal, tea and toast with cooked food being available when desired. On a number of occasions patients awoke later in the morning (10.30 hours) but were still able to take breakfast, which was ordered over the telephone and served by a member of the kitchen staff in the patient's own room. During the morning, the medical director invariably made her presence known to various patients and staff, going in to see patients, carrying out physical examinations and chatting generally to patients and relatives alike, in a quiet, unassuming way, that I had not personally experienced before. The medical director made no attempt to seek nurses to act as a chaperone or assist with patient examinations, unless it was necessary (for example where the patient needed moving). It was reassuring to see this type of unobtrusive approach adopted by all the medical staff who also appeared to go out of their way to seek advice and information from nurses.

The patient day was punctuated, by the arrival of the lunchtime meal trolley. Lunch comprising three courses was invariably taken in the patient's own room. Visiting relatives were invited to have lunch in the dining room with the patient if they wished. The quality of food was very good and in particular, because of the short distance it travelled, was always hot. Patients chose their own food and were able to change their minds and have other food if they felt unable to eat that which they previously ordered. After patients had taken their lunch, staff went for theirs, one group before and one after the 13.00 hours early/late shift handover.

Summoning nurse assistance

A noticeable feature of nursing work at the Beeches was the almost constant use of nurse call buttons. These inter-communication systems were in each room and when patients were in bed, chair, bathroom or toilet, the call button was always placed in a readily accessible position for both patient and/or relatives to summon assistance from nurses. It became a feature of day to day work at the hospice that, at any time, nurses could be answering a call when the 'buzzer' goes off. During the day nurses were not allowed to mute the sound of the 'buzzer', which was often heard throughout the unit. The caller was identified via a wall-mounted electronic display board behind the nurses' station, together with an illuminated light outside the patient's room. Some nurses left patients on the toilet, requesting that they 'buzzed' for assistance when ready, so they could then go back to the nurses' station and await the call. At other times assistance was summoned for a variety of reasons, from getting up to go to the toilet, to requesting pain relief. The sound of buzzers going off became a central feature of the nursing work at the Beeches throughout the day.

During the morning several patients went to the day hospice for coffee, or to chat and just see what was going on. Highly dependent patients were able to go outside in their beds when the weather was fine. There do not appear to be limits placed on what patients are able to do which includes shopping, visiting the pub or merely going for a walk. The Beeches facilitated patients who wished to go round the grounds in a wheel chair (which I offered to do on several occasions due to the nice weather and the appealing environment of the hospice grounds). This was in stark contrast to hospital settings, where the patient's day was largely determined by the needs of the hospital and those providing patient care, notwithstanding however, many patients in hospital were admitted for treatment, whereas most patients at the Beeches attended for respite care, medical assessment and, above all, rest.

Afternoon and evening

Unlike my research in hospital, the pace of work at the hospice remained fairly constant during the afternoon, as nurses attempted to make no deliberate effort towards achieving their work goals by lunchtime. This meant that in the afternoon there was still plenty of 'work' to do. The afternoons were a popular visiting time for relatives and friends, who invariably wished to chat to members of the care team, with nurses in particular taking the opportunity to get to know patients' families. Interestingly what hospital nurses perceived as nursing work in terms of any physical patient care activity, was not shared by staff at the Beeches. The administration of drugs, which was an important nursing activity, took place mid-morning and mid-afternoon. Patients were however always given drugs to relieve pain and symptoms when needed outside of the afore-mentioned scheduled times. Social activity, such as taking a patient out or playing cards was considered an appropriate activity for nurses and anything that included a patient, such as applying make-up or merely sitting and chatting was perceived as a very legitimate part of nursing work. Patients' birthdays were always celebrated with cakes ordered from the hospice kitchen, to supplement the food and drink brought by relatives. Patients and in some cases relatives, were able to leave food and drink for patients in the ward 'fridge, including special dietary foods and alcohol.

Afternoon and early evening activity was similarly punctuated by the evening meal, which once again comprised three courses, being served from a trolley and taken in the patient's room. After the evening meal, visitors appeared in greater numbers with the late shift nurses spending time with patients and their families and the nurse call 'buzzers' playing a significant part in summoning help throughout the evening. Some patients retired to bed early before the night staff arrived, just lying in bed watching television with their visitors who could and commonly did stay until after the night staff came on duty.

The pace of work

The most significant issue relating to hospice and hospital resources was the staffing ratios. In the hospice the patient:staff ratio was often 3:1 compared with my hospital data, which indicated a 7:1 ratio. This has a major impact not only on the way care was provided but also the pace at which nurses worked. I had tremendous difficulty getting used to the slow pace of work in the hospice and relative lack of urgency in the way nurses performed nursing care. My previous experiences in hospital meant that I had to work at a fast pace, in order to be able to meet the needs of all the allocated patients in my care and to be able to complete all the perceived work. Whilst this approach was not always made explicit by hospital nurses, it was clear that at least during the morning shift periods, many hospital wards were considered to experience '*the rush hour*', with nurses (often understaffed) attempting to get as much of the 'work' done as possible during the morning shift which included getting patients washed, dressed and ready for a range of activities such as medical ward rounds and out-patient clinic appointments (Costello 2000).

At the Beeches I was eager to start my participant observation and become part of the nursing team by carrying out tasks such as changing bedding and generally hurrying about carrying out practical tasks such as emptying commodes. Ultimately I became aware that it was not necessary to rush around as I and a colleague only had two or three patients to look after and two of the patients were still asleep! Moreover, much of the nursing work pivoted on the patients' wishes, for example one morning having prepared a bath for a patient, I arrived back only to find that he had changed his mind and decided to go back to sleep! I asked nurses at the Beeches who had previously worked on busy medical wards in NHS Trust Hospitals, how they found the pace when they first started? Kirsty (Staff Nurse) pointed out that:

> At first, it was very different and a bit difficult to get used to, mainly because of the numbers of staff and patients, after a while, you tend to think what's the rush, why do I need to work at such a pace, here it's the patient who sets the pace not the staff.

Initially, the Beeches appeared to have no explicit ward routine around which much nursing care in modern hospices was reportedly organised (Field & James 1993). It soon became evident that the pace and routine was structured by patients and their ability or otherwise, to do what they needed to do. Many patients once up and dressed, chose to stay in their rooms where they watched television, listened to the radio or read papers. Patients rarely ventured into the lounges (one for smokers and one for non-smokers). Similarly, I did not see anyone ever make use of the multi-faith room. These observations were consistent with those made of patients in hospital who tended to restrict themselves to their bedside. This was often for practical reasons, as they were unable to mobilise well enough or were afraid to walk too far unassisted.

Caring for poorly patients

Despite the slower pace of work and the focus placed on patients' choice and personal preference, nursing work at the Beeches was often busy with nurses working extremely hard, especially during periods of high patient dependency and when staff shortages occurred. One particular period stands out because of the large number of poorly patients who were not in a position to use the nurse call 'buzzers'. This created the effect of making the unit seem eerily quiet since I had become used to 'buzzers' constantly going off. This gave the impression that the unit was indeed very busy. In reality, it was when the 'buzzers' were not sounding that nurses were working their hardest, caring for highly dependent poorly patients (many of whom were in the advanced stages of dying) and all needing close and sensitive terminal care. During such times, the unit would be very quiet and the nurses were not to be seen outside of patients' rooms.

When a number of patients were dying or highly dependent, nurses spent long periods of time with them and their family in their rooms. Volunteers manned the nursing station, answered the telephone and became reluctant to take nurses away from the bedside. Acting as ward clerks they would inform visitors that the patient was receiving nursing care and ask that families and relatives wait in the reception area until they were ready to receive them. It was important to do this when patients were poorly, as relatives were not always aware of the impending nature of the patient's death. Much of the nursing work at the Beeches in situations like this is based on psychological nursing care, the effectiveness of such care being largely based on nurses' interpersonal skills together with their knowledge of and relationship with the patient and their family.

Staff morale

Nursing work in a hospice carries with it a number of challenges that impinge on the morale of staff, least of all the stress of managing highly dependent patients facing impending death. It is not suprising that an abundance of literature has accumulated which identifies the extent to which nurses working in such settings tend to experience varying degrees of stress (Vachon 1987).

One of the notable features of all the staff in the Beeches was their sustained high level of morale despite, at times, working below their established staffing levels for a prolonged period which resulted from the G grade sister leaving and not being replaced. Despite the significance of this change, nurses openly discussed the loss of their leader and pondered on who would replace her. Staff morale was an important aspect of hospice care and seemed to be helped by not allowing the level of work to exceed the available resources. Interestingly, during the time when staff numbers were low admissions did not reach full capacity. This seemed to help the staff cope with the workload. One strategy successfully employed by staff to maintain their morale was to organise social occasions, which helped team integration and provided topics for discussion and much essential gossip! There appeared to be genuine concern shown for the welfare of individual staff members that was not as evident in the hospital ward studies. The staff group as a whole were integrated in a number of ways; there being a willingness to listen and share ideas, irrespective of which member of staff expressed the view and no discernible overt inter-team rivalry!

Teamwork and nursing work

Closely related to the notably high staff morale levels was the cohesion of the nurses when working together in teams. Since the 1970s, the professional ideology of nursing work has focused attention on teamwork as a way of delivering effective nursing care (Evers 1981). This approach influenced by industrial work production models, sought to maximise the use of available resources, by enabling one or two qualified nurses to form two teams of subordinates available to patients. The origin of teamwork derived from the emphasis placed upon efficiency in the NHS in the 1980s and the adoption of scientific management models by 'new-wave' management structures. From these came the devolution of decision making to form semi-autonomous team structures. Efficiency focused on the responsiveness of the team to the patient, with success measured in terms of patient or customer satisfaction, as well as hospital output. Nurses perceived that working as part of a team ensured that organisational goals were more readily achieved, thus making them more personally effective in the workplace. The heavy demands placed on health care workers, as a result of increases in throughput of patients, arising from political pressures, ensures more patients are treated in a shorter time. In essence the popular notion of teamwork suggests that each team member contributes different skills to nursing care, which enriches the collective process (Shukla 1982). Teamwork involves groups of nurses collectively working towards the accomplishment of specific tasks, being a feature of nursing work in a variety of forms and integral to the work of nurses in both UK hospitals and hospices. This ideology meets the needs of patients as well as the perceived hospice philosophy, which is set out in the mission statement (see Figure 4.1). More recently however, evidence suggests that the dynamics of teamwork in hospital are changing as a result of changes in nurses' roles. With the development of Clinical Nurse Specialists (CNSs) and nurse consultants, medical staff in hospital are no longer dominating teams and their power over nurses appears to be diminishing (Booth et al 2003).

The organisation of nursing work at the Beeches was based on nurses working in two teams during the day (Blue and Green), with night staff achieving their goals collectively, through working as one team. It should be stressed that day shift working was quite different to that on the night shift where there was a far lower complement of nurses. Nurses on night duty often looked after individual patients on their own whilst working with colleagues collectively as part of one team, but this in no way detracted from the notion and principles of teamwork. One of the prominent features of the observation and interview data from the Beeches, was that much of the nursing work took place as a result of nurses working together and by communicating their individual efforts to other members of the team.

Nursing teamwork according to Waters (1987) involves those nurses on day shifts constituting teams and working to achieve their practical and organisational goals by working together. At the Beeches each team was led by either an F grade sister or an E grade staff nurse, assisted by D grade staff nurses and HSWs (who formed the unqualified nursing component). The allocation of patients to each team was often rather arbitrary, in many cases prior to a patient's admission and commonly based on equitable allocation of staff to each team as well as in recognition of the patient's level of dependency. The teamwork structures were notional rather than fixed and depended largely on the number of staff available for each shift. Team members from the Blue and Green teams often working together, although invariably respective team members attempted to keep to their own teams, when staffing levels permitted. This was also a feature of the researcher's hospital experience with team nursing, although teams in hospital invariably did not function according to the teamwork rhetoric (Costello 2000), whereas at the Beeches the teams did invariably work in the anticipated way with qualified nurses and HSWs working collectively as teams.

Case study

The following case study depicts what I consider to be a typical patient from the Beeches who was admitted for 2-week routine respite care. George Connors was a 78 year old man with cancer of the bowel, having had a colostomy (stoma) several months previously, which was not functioning properly due to the presence of another tumour. He also had an in-welling urinary catheter in situ. George was admitted as a result of his GPs referral for respite care. The aim of the admission was twofold. First, to relieve the burden of care on his wife (Ethel) who was 72 years of age and suffered from arthritis. Ethel was finding it difficult to lift George in and out of bed. Secondly, by admitting George, it was possible to assess his symptom management to avoid any preventable complications arising whilst he was at home. The couple had one son Sean, aged 46 years, and three grandchildren. The family were considered close with Sean visiting regularly. George never complained about any aspect of the care he received and was considered a popular, cheerful and well-mannered patient who was also quite deaf. His wife Ethel came in to see him every day spending between 5 and 6 hours at the hospice. She brought fresh pyjamas that she insisted he wear during the day. George gave the impression that this was the way he was supposed to behave when he was in the hospice. During his stay he developed a urinary tract infection, which was treated successfully with antibiotics and following the administration of suppositories and an enema, his stoma began to function properly. George also developed a small sacral sore which was treated and responded well to pressure area care. Ethel was asked to see the hospice social worker, who was able to secure attendance allowance for her and a much increased level of home-care aid together with district nurse and occupational therapy support. When George was admitted Ethel received very little help with her husband's welfare, other than home-care aid twice each week.

George was discharged home after his 2-week stay, having undergone a thorough assessment, which had enabled his wife to enjoy a well-earned rest and the opportunity of far more support, in an attempt at assisting her with the care of George. This included additional home lifting aids, as a result of a risk assessment that was carried out during his stay at the Beeches and recommended that Ethel should not be involved in as much manual handling as she had been undertaking prior to his admission.

Reflections on the case study
This brief case study depicted a typical patient admitted to the Beeches and was a deliberate attempt to convey to the reader that, despite being a place where many patients are terminally ill, the hospice also provides care for many patients who stay a short time and go home with an increased quality of life. George was the type of patient the Beeches was keen to admit. Although not privy to the referral data or to details of which patients were admitted, I was told that there was always a bed available for patients whose relatives required respite care. This was locally referred to as a respite care bed. Equally during the time of the study the hospice was only fully occupied on one occasion and that only lasted a few days. The hospice was keen to promote the view that, like many modern hospices, the Beeches was not a place where patients came to die. Many patients died after their admission to the hospice

although (at the time of their admission) this was not anticipated. It would appear therefore that there was an unwritten policy which identified that the hospice would have bed(s) available as much as possible for people in a similar position to George. This is an interesting and less well-known feature of modern hospice care. Although as Eve & Smith (1996) point out, the average length of stay of a hospice patient in the UK is 12–14 days. There is likely to be tremendous variance in the length of stay of hospice patients, which will depend on a number of factors such as the size of the hospice and the number of staff working there. George was admitted at a time when there were a number of patients who were rather poorly and he was in a double room where the patient in the next bed (Ken) died. Ken was very ill when he was moved into George's room and was frequently receiving attention from the nurses. Ken's death was dealt with in the usual quiet and efficient manner, but as Honeybun et al (1992) point out hospice care is not without a number of difficulties for patients. Their study outlined some of the adverse effects of being in a hospice and sharing in the grief when fellow patients die. George did not however express any undue concern when Ken died. In reality, the two of them had little social contact. George was regarded as a quiet unassuming individual who did not openly engage in social interaction with others except the staff and his family who visited regularly. The two of them had little to do with each other, partly because of George's deafness, which was a handicap in enabling him to converse easily with others. Ken was also not in a position to engage in much social discourse outside of his own family. George, who was aware that Ken was terminally ill, judging by the amount of nursing attention he received and the extent of his many physical needs, perhaps shared my observations of Ken's situation. On reflection, it should perhaps be pointed out that the patient's perception (and that of some health care professionals) is that a hospice is a place where patients come to die. To a certain extend this is accurate, although as George was told before his admission, the primary reason he came into the Beeches was to enable his wife to have a rest. Hockley (1997:85) points out that:

> Generally a patient coming to a hospice would be expected to have less than three months to live.

The case study of George reflects the modern hospice approach to palliative care by embracing the notion of caring for both the patient and the family. Hospice patients gain significant benefits from hospice care. George had a very enjoyable stay in the Beeches:

> I can honestly say that it's been great in here, I've been well looked after, and my wife has had a well earned break from all the work involved in looking after me, well I feel champion, you can put that in yer book if you like.

Reflecting on George's stay at the Beeches, it is clear that palliative care for patients in a hospice should include the care of the family and the provision of respite care is a clear tangible expression of such care.

Summary

This chapter has given an overview and some insights into the organisation and provision of nursing care in a hospice context. The chapter has thrown into relief the link between palliative care and hospice ideology, in terms of patient-centredness and the development of what is called a 'holistic family orientated' framework. Whilst many hospital nurses may subscribe to this philosophy, it is clear from earlier chapters that, in practice, much nursing care in hospitals derives from a desire to meet organisational not patients' needs. The structures in hospice, i.e. the limited (but reliance on) medical intervention and the different type of relationships between doctors and nurses, make a significant impact on the way care is planned and provided. In general terms nurses enjoy greater autonomy in hospices and medical staff tend to adopt a more low profile position compared with their hospital counterparts. It should be borne in mind that each hospice will have its own unique variations in organisational culture. Medical staff at the Beeches had a much more focused role in terms of prescribing medication and conducting medical assessments. Whilst they became involved in a wide range of activity, their role was limited due to their time commitments and the ability of nurses to effectively manage the patient care. This differs from the hospital care described in the previous chapters, which was largely based on the biomedical model of care; which placed the patient's condition and treatment above the values of the patient and their family. In terms of physical structures, it is also clear that hospices have greater material and human resources at their disposal and the patient : nurse ratio is much lower. This enables nurses to provide a more personal and individualised care. Hospice nurses at times, still perceive themselves to be under pressure and over worked just like their hospital colleagues because they are often able to set their targets much higher than nurses in other contexts. It may be argued that the prevailing culture, structural processes and material advantages of hospices enable them to provide higher standards of care.

This chapter and the previous three have highlighted the importance of teamwork and the importance of developing positive relations between patients and staff. Effective teamwork helps to improve staff morale, at least when there are sufficient numbers to call a team! In both hospital and hospice contexts, external constraints such as staff shortages negatively influence the quality of nursing care. Moreover, the structural aspects of care in terms of how well members of the team work together and the harmony between their respective roles, plays a part in the provision of good care in any context. Tension and friction between team members can at times be as destructive as insufficient staff numbers, as cohesive staff who work well together can compensate in the short term for a dysfunctional team that may be experiencing a difficult time developing teamwork.

In Chapter 5 next, a critical analysis is made of the nursing practices in both hospital and hospice contexts. This chapter considers the psychological care of patients in both hospital and hospice as emotional labour and also reviews the notion as to whether hospices do indeed medicalise death and dying. Chapter 5 considers the degree to which hospice principles can be incorporated into hospital care. In particular the chapter will consider a range of ideas which surround hospice care by examining the ways that are being used to try to improve standards of palliative care in hospitals and the problems and successes that nurses and doctors have encountered.

Further reading

Costello J. (1994) 'The role of the nurse in the multi-disciplinary team'. *Reviews in Clinical Gerontology* 4, 169–76.

This article is a literature review focused on the major works and research studies on multi-disciplinary teamworking. The article is largely based on nurses working in elderly care settings although much of the discussion is aimed at nurses and doctors working and, in most cases, not working well together in hospital contexts. It provides a useful overview of the literature in the area but will need to be updated to keep the reader aware of contemporary literature and the changes in teamworking within different settings.

Johnson I.S., Rogers R., Biswas B. & Ahmedzai S. (1990) 'What do hospices do? A survey of hospices in the United Kingdom'. *British Medical Journal* 300, 24 March, 791–93.

This original research study examined clinical activity in 98 hospices in the UK and collected data on clinical activity using questionnaires sent to matrons/senior sisters. The findings indicate that in those hospices with full time medical directors throughput was greater and more patients had palliative surgery and became organ donors than those without full time medical cover. The authors point out that responses from hospices with full time consultants were more likely to refer to the hospice in technical terms such as pain relief centres than those without full time medical staff. The article is interesting in that it reveals the perceptions of hospice nurses based on the influence of medical staff as well as the increasing medicalisation of certain hospices.

Parkes C.M. & Parkes J. (1984) ' "Hospice" versus "hospital" care – re-evaluation after 10 years as seen by surviving spouses'. *Post-graduate Medical Journal* 60, 120–24.

This article written by the famous Psychiatrist and his wife reports on a study comparing hospice (St Christopher's) and hospital terminal care in 1967–69 with care in 1977–79. The study points out that patients and carers reported less personal stress in both settings in the later study and it is believed that patients experienced less pain. The success of the later studies is attributed to advances in training in terminal care.

Payne S., Hillier R., Langley-Evans A. & Roberts T. (1996) 'Impact of witnessing death on hospice patients'. *Social Science and Medicine* 43, 12, 1785–94.

This academic article reports on a research study conducted by the authors. The article discusses a number of wide-ranging issues which the reader may find useful when analysing the impact that hospice care has had on the management of dying patients in a number of settings. The introduction highlights the contemporary role of hospices and the advances they have made in relation to meeting the needs of dying patients and their families. The discussion on information control and awareness of dying represents a good review of the earlier work of Glaser & Strauss (1965). The study reports on a well controlled piece of research whose findings suggest that knowing about impending death and witnessing death in a hospice are not necessarily indicative of distress measured in terms of depression.

Saunders C. (1996) 'A personal therapeutic journey'. *British Medical Journal* 313, 21–28 December, 1599–601.

This is a very informative and moving article which traces the developments made in the early years of Cecily Saunders' career, and identifies the progress made in what has become the foundation of modern hospice care. The article discusses active care, total pain control and the family as a unit of care and is written from a personal perspective.

Seale C.F. (1989) 'What happens in hospices? A review of research evidence'. *Social Science and Medicine* 28(6), 551–59.

This rather excellent review traces the origins of the modern hospice movement and compares hospital and hospice models of care. Seale highlights key differences and similarities between hospitals and hospices. He suggests that hospital staff have learnt from the work of hospice nurses although there are key areas where hospice models of care differ from hospital approaches. It is a very interesting critical analysis that provides sound evidence supporting the view that hospice care is similar to hospital nursing care.

5

Improving care for dying patients in hospital

Introduction

Palliative care is rapidly emerging as an integrated part of health care delivery. This is due partly to the parlous state of terminal care for dying patients in acute hospital settings (discussed in Chapter 1) and also because of the need to improve palliative care for dying patients, which has become apparent in the UK through a number of publications. These begin with the recommendations of the Calman & Hine report (1995), which highlighted the view that optimal care for cancer patients can only be achieved if the services are linked to a comprehensive cancer care system. More recently, the need to consider ways to improve standards in hospital care was further underlined by the Government's NHS *Cancer Care Plan* (Department of Health 2000) which points out that:

> Providing the best possible care for dying patients remains of paramount importance. Too many patients still experience distressing symptoms, poor nursing care, poor psychological and social support and inadequate communication from health care professionals durng the final stages of their illness.

Traditionally, hospitals have largely focused attention on acute care with the aim of ensuring quality and often prolongation of life. Increasingly however, with advances in medical science in general and health care in particular, more and more people are spending a considerable amount of time living with a life threatening medical illness. The purpose of this chapter is to examine some of the difficulties associated with bringing about change in hospitals by looking at organisational culture, ideology and some of the problems associated with facilitating innovation. In doing this, the chapter will reflect on some of the problems associated with the provision of care for dying patients within institutional contexts, describing developments that have taken place for improving palliative care and comparing these with the relative 'gold standard' of hospice settings.

The chapter focuses on ways in which the quality of life can be measured and assessed as well as looking at a specific way in which hospice principles can be incorporated into hospitals, through the use of Hospital Based Specialist Palliative Care Teams (HBSPCTs) whose aim is to import hospice principles and practice such as pain and symptom control into hospitals. Secondly the chapter examines, the way in which hospitals have attempted to improve nursing care through the use of Integrated Care Pathways (ICPs) for the dying. The aim of these tools is to assist in monitoring and documenting patient progress and to support assessment, planning and effective intervention (Ellershaw & Wilkinson 2003). Both of these approaches will be described and evaluated in relation to the way they can be used to improve the patient's quality of life and for the contribution they make to communicating the provision of palliative care to other members of the multi-disciplinary team.

Palliative care and terminal care

In the past many professional practitioners in hospital, have been criticised for providing poor standards of terminal care. A major challenge to improving the care to dying patients is changing their attitude and adopting a palliative care ideology. A fundamental step towards this is to recognise that terminal care is an important (albeit one part of) providing palliation for patients with life threatening medical conditions. For some nurses and doctors, the care of dying patients is encapsulated within the euphemism of TLC, often used in patient's notes to signify that the patient is to be 'kept comfortable' and that 'active forms of treatment' are to be avoided. The values being expressed in the 'terminal care passivity' are often well meaning, but prevent nurses from reaching out and recognising that the patient is living before they die. In extreme cases, decisions can be made about the care of the patient such as determining that they are not to be resuscitated, receive blood transfusions or intravenous fluids.

Enshrined within the notion of terminal care is the emphasis on ensuring that the physical aspects of care are well maintained and the patient is kept symptom free, clean, dry and prevented from developing complications of their condition such as pressure sores. Despite being important issues, in some cases they may become the only care aims and therefore, limit and prevent palliative care from being more patient focused. Evidence from studies of palliative care nursing supports the view that nurses and others place great emphasis on physical aspects of care, with much less attention given to psychological aspects of care such as spiritual comfort (James 1986, Field 1989, Costello 2000, Hopkinson 2002).

Another limitation of terminal care is that it often fails to see the importance of support for family and friends of the dying person. The latter is an integral part of palliative care, which many nurses feel is as *important* as the care given to the patient in terms of preventing later adverse grief reactions. In many ways therefore, changing standards of care for the dying in hospital requires nurses to change their approach and consider that the dying are also the living and that whilst difficult to determine, the quality of the patient's last days of life should be maximised and determined by the needs of the patient and their loved ones. All too often, as Chapters 1 and 2 have outlined, patients' needs in hospital take second place to those of the organisation. Implementing palliative care principles also involves looking at the constraints placed on providing effective care by the organisational culture in which care takes place.

Patients as customers

Against the backdrop to the *new modern dependable NHS*, many hospital administrators would argue that, the business culture of hospital trusts requires the organisation to become receptive to the needs of the consumer. Patients are perceived as customers and are therefore now being asked what they want, whether they are satisfied with care and audited as to their level of dependency and the degree of risk they and nurses are being exposed to. During the series of changes that have taken place in the last decade the roles of hospital staff have radically altered. Most notably the power wielded by the medical profession has been curtailed as a result of increasing specialisation, segregation and fragmentation of services. A senior doctor in a local hospice who retired from the NHS summarised the medical perspective by pointing out that '… these days doctors often perceive themselves to be technicians who are at the beck and call of hospital administrators'. Despite a number of innovations taking place in hospitals such as Hospital Based Specialist Palliative Care Teams and the introduction of Integrated Care Pathways for the dying, little evidence exists that standards of care have improved. Moreover, it may be argued that with the increasing throughput of patients, there are now even more challenges facing nurses who may wish to adopt a new perspective on caring for dying patients.

Palliative care in hospital

There are a number of reasons why palliative care is such a major challenge to hospital staff. First, nurses working in hospitals experience much greater variance in terms of the type of dying patients they encounter. In the A&E department for example the sudden death of a baby brought in by distressed parents takes place at the same time as a sudden road traffic accident victim dies. In the elderly care unit the dying patient may require several weeks of intensive care, whilst on renal units and in specialist areas like the CCU and ICU death is a regular occurrence. Staff reactions to individual deaths also vary according to the context in which death takes place. The relief and sense of release felt following the death of a very 'poorly patient' who had lingered for some time contrasts with the life saving interventions made in the Special Care Baby Unit (SCBU), where death may be seen as a failure. In these instances, age is an influential factor. The death of an elderly patient appears to be accepted much more readily than the death of a child, which reflects cultural changes towards death and dying in the UK. Hospitals manage death on a wide and diverse scale despite the way in which they attempt to sequestrate death from the wards by attempting to hide the deceased from view after death. Unexpected deaths resulting from road traffic accidents and traumatic deaths due to suicide are often tainted by trauma. At the same time the increasing number of deaths from strokes and cardiac arrests (the largest cause of death in the UK), make death a familiar feature within many hospitals. In modern times, a patient's 'dying trajectory' is often unique and individualised. Many patients are treated with powerful chemotherapeutic agents and radiation therapy, which have the potential to cause distressing side effects, and despite these treatments patients then face impending death.

Incorporating hospice principles into hospitals

Hospitals are busy places where communication problems and the mismanagement of information concerning terminal diagnosis regularly take place (Field & Copp 1999). A number of classic papers on staff stress and morale such as Revans' study (1974) point out that *'hospitals are cradled in anxiety'*. Such issues are made more difficult due to increasing specialisation, segregation and fragmentation of services. A fundamental difference between the Beeches and the hospital wards described in Chapter 1 is the input (admission), throughput (length of stay) and output (discharge) of patients. The use of such terminology reflects the language of the business culture and helps to denote that many hospitals have developed a business culture. The statistical evidence clearly demonstrates the comparative differences between hospitals with high turnovers and a very diverse range of patients and hospices with relatively small numbers and invariably one disease. Figures 5.1 and 5.2 illustrate this point by demonstrating the admission and discharge of patients to the hospice and hospital respectively for one quarter.

In a comparative sense, the statistics for the Beeches are similar to those for the same quarter 3 years earlier in one ward of the hospital study (see Chapter 1). The ward figures reflect the differences in the number of admissions, length of stay and deaths. As you would expect, the hospice dealt with more deaths despite having fewer in-patient beds (12), but the number of patients passing through the hospice (throughput) was also very different. More revealing are the staff ratios. The total staff numbers for both areas (night and day shifts) at the Beeches (24 staff) and the hospital ward (13) show the inverse relationship between the two in terms of staff numbers and patient throughput.

Admitted to in-patient unit	89
Average length of stay (in days)	17
Numbers of deaths	52
Total number of nurses	24

Figure 5.1   The Beeches: admissions, length of stay and deaths
1 January–31 March 2001

*Average age of patients admitted to the in-patient unit was 69
with the youngest being 37 and the oldest 93.*

Admitted	121
Numbers of deaths	24
Discharges	97
Average length of stay (in days)	27
Total number of nurses	13

Figure 5.2   Hospital admissions and discharges
1 January–31 March 1998

Hospital and hospice care

A number of studies comparing hospital and hospice care have
highlighted the contrasting features of each setting. Many
have focused attention on the views of surviving spouses (Parkes
1978, Parkes & Parkes 1984, Seale & Kelly 1997). The findings
highlight some of the more well known comparative features such
as the amount of information provided about dying which was
found to be higher in hospices (Seale & Kelly 1997). Parkes &
Parkes (1984) found that pain and distress had reduced in hospice
and hospital patients when they compared data from their earlier
study in 1967 to one 10 years later. They also found that in the

later study patients' spouses reported feeling more anxiety and had less involvement in care within hospital, but felt closer to staff in the hospice than in hospital. These studies demonstrate two things. First, that palliative care for many people is improving, although, it seems that hospices have higher standards of care than hospitals. Second, it would seem that most practitioners working in hospitals and hospices acknowledge that palliative care is not an optional extra provided to certain patients, but should be an integral and important core element of the nursing care for dying patients.

Individual care: rhetoric and reality

One of the central features of palliative care is the development of an individualised approach to patient care, which despite the rhetoric is difficult to achieve in hospitals, due largely to the 'production model' approach being utilised. Saunders' (1970) quote *'you matter because you are you, we will help you live until you die'* reflects one of the fundamental features of palliative care, namely that the individual patient and their needs are paramount and above the needs of the organisation. One of the contrasting features of my research in hospice and hospital was the way in which hospices and their staff actually served the patient. An example of this was the way in which the hospice routine was determined by the needs of the patient. When a patient woke up they would invariably have their breakfast when they were ready. In contrast, hospital routine such as the times of waking and sleeping were rigidly enforced by the staff who all seemed to be clear about what constituted the rules. Many of these, such as the times of meals, medication and visiting hours were closely adhered to.

Secondly, effective palliative care requires the provision of support to the family and friends of the patient who are involved in and in some cases help to determine the aims and outcomes of care and treatment. Once again hospitals have a very poor history of involving families in care, although there is evidence that this is changing, often doctors and nurses focus their attention exclusively on the patient. Thirdly, palliative care at least in hospices, actively involves other members of the multi-disciplinary team as a key component. This is a problematic issue in hospital contexts since despite the rhetoric, nurses and other professionals in hospital are largely dictated to by their medical colleagues (Evers 1981, Hill 1998).

The differences between hospitals and hospices are often very clear, hospitals were built for different purposes and function differently. Although it is easy to identify and criticise the lack of care for certain groups of patients, it should be borne in mind that hospitals cater for everyone, irrespective of their medical condition, on a 24 hour basis. Bearing this in mind, it is perhaps not difficult to see why people from other countries, who are often very impressed by the health care system in the UK revere the British NHS. In a contextual sense, hospitals are complex structures where issues of power being wielded by dominant groups mainly medical staff, become a key issue in decision making. The influence of biomedical approaches is one of the major features of hospital culture. Treatment regimes, hospital routine policy making and ideological influence permeate the fibre of hospital life. Nurses, as the major occupational group, despite their collective power, often act in a subordinate way towards medical staff (Mackay 1993). The structure of medical teams or 'firms' is helpful in perpetuating the hierarchical structure. Junior doctors are often afraid to voice an opinion that may be viewed negatively by their consultant (Lawler 1991, Costello 2000). It is only in what Klein (1998) calls '*the new politics of the NHS*' that a different type of command comes into play, wearing suits and using technology to exercise authority over medical staff. Despite the increasing pressure to work in teams, there is no clear evidence that medical staff are able to work in a way conducive towards effective multi-disciplinary teamwork because of the often entrenched way in which they have become used to and expect compliance from other professional groups (Ovretveit 1995). In other contexts such as nursing homes, there is evidence of nurses managing patient care and making decisions with doctors (GPs) and patients, in a setting that is much less hierarchical (see Chapter 6).

I now wish to turn to two innovations which have been adopted in an attempt to bring about improvements in the care of dying patients in hospitals. These are the introduction of Hospital Based Specialist Palliative Care Teams and the adoption of Integrated Care Pathways. Both of these measures being used today in the NHS have made an impact on palliative care, although it should be pointed out that their progress continues to be evaluated and in some cases critical evaluation of the precise role they play in improving care is yet to be determined.

Hospital Based Specialist Palliative Care Teams

The question of whether hospice principles can be introduced into hospitals is problematic. In practice, as the preceding sections have highlighted, introducing new ideas and implementing change in hospitals requires a good deal of effort, not only by specialist teams who facilitate change, but also by hospital practitioners, managers and administrators. One of the most effective ways of developing palliative care in hospitals has been through the introduction of Hospital Based Specialist Palliative Care Teams (HBSPCTs). This approach which began at St Thomas's Hospital in 1976 was initiated by a combination of the need to improve care for patients with life threatening medical conditions, as well as by policy initiatives (Department of Health (DoH) 1987). In themselves, these initiatives were, in part, a response to adverse criticism of the poor standards of terminal care in hospital highlighted in the literature, as well as a need to manage the palliative care of patients more effectively. Recent records show there to be over 380 teams in the UK (Ellershaw 2001). Many are referred to as *Macmillan support services* (reflecting the predominance of this group) as well as *symptom control teams* and are often viewed as being advisory in nature. Many teams established in the 1980s consisted of two or more Macmillan nurses who together with secretarial support developed medical input from local anaesthetists and hospital physicians. In some hospitals this type of support may consist of one Clinical Nurse Specialist and in others the team may consist of doctors, nurses, social workers and chaplains. Clark & Seymour (1999) argue that the arrival of doctors and nurses in hospitals, whose role was to focus on palliative care, arose from public recognition of the success of the hospice movement. The emergence of HBSPCTs has also been influenced by outside sources, chiefly in the form of large charities such as Macmillan Cancer Relief who play a pivotal role in 'pump priming' the funding of specialist nurses to form the basis of many of the early teams. The Macmillan strategy of providing initial funding for 3 years gave impetus for their growth throughout the UK (see Booth et al 2003).

The role of HBSPCTs

The precise role of the HBSPC team is determined locally according to the pre-existing knowledge of nurses and doctors about the problems they face as well as their resources, local culture, and the success of the particular team in establishing links with their medical and nursing colleagues. HBSPCTs often consist of several health care professionals and in some cases a specialist in medical palliative care often on a part-time basis. Referrals come from all ward areas but patients invariably have a cancer diagnosis. Patients are referred to specialist teams via hospital doctors with the majority of referrals being based on requests for pain control (Ellershaw 2001). Figure 5.3 illustrates some of the questions and considerations made when making a referral to an HBSPCT.

The aim of such teams is twofold: first to support the patient and carers to improve the quality of life from the time of diagnosis up to and including bereavement (NCHSPCS 1996). Second to offer support to professional carers who, because of a range of organisational issues, are unable to meet the specific demands of the patient. In practice this is a complex task that involves the coordination of care to patients in hospital with palliative care needs, with a focus on alleviating pain and suffering. Often team members become very involved in educating nursing and medical staff into ways of providing a more effective pattern of care to patients, many of whom face impending death. The notion of 'the team' is slightly disingenuous since, in many cases teams consist of two nurses and/or a part-time physician. Their role in hospital has been largely educational because they are so small. They have never found it easy to cover a wide geographic area and their ability to disseminate advice and influence care has been hampered by medical dominance (Clark & Seymour 1999), lack of resources and organisation (Kite 1997) and a range of organisational and political constraints (The National Council for Hospice and Specialist Palliative Care Services 1996). The function of HBSPCTs is to:

- Provide advice to professionals without a patient referral.
- Conduct an assessment of a particular patient and offer advice about future treatment and care.
- Carry out short term intervention as requested by a specific group of physicians or ward based staff.

```
┌─────────────────────────────────────────────────────────────┐
│          Does the patient have cancer or is in the            │
│             terminal phase of a life threatening              │
│                     medical illness?                          │
└─────────────────────────────────────────────────────────────┘
                             YES
                              ↓
┌─────────────────────────────────────────────────────────────┐
│        Does the patient have specialist palliative care       │
│           needs not met by the primary carers?                │
└─────────────────────────────────────────────────────────────┘

       If discharge is planned ALL these patients must be
        referred to district nurses for assessment.
                             YES
                              ↓
┌─────────────────────────────────────────────────────────────┐
│            Is the patient aware of the diagnosis?             │
└─────────────────────────────────────────────────────────────┘

                             YES
                              ↓
┌─────────────────────────────────────────────────────────────┐
│   Does the patient/carer want to see a specialist palliative  │
│                         care nurse?                           │
└─────────────────────────────────────────────────────────────┘

                             YES
                              ↓
┌─────────────────────────────────────────────────────────────┐
│               What is the reason for referral?               │
└─────────────────────────────────────────────────────────────┘

                              ↓
┌─────────────────────────────────────────────────────────────┐
│   Symptom control, psychosocial care, help and support for    │
│        the carer future specialist care for the patient       │
└─────────────────────────────────────────────────────────────┘

                              ↓
┌─────────────────────────────────────────────────────────────┐
│  Referral assessed and discussed with primary carers. Needs   │
│  assessed at level of intervention required from palliative   │
│                        care services                          │
└─────────────────────────────────────────────────────────────┘

                              ↓
┌─────────────────────────────────────────────────────────────┐
│                   Assessment visit arranged                   │
└─────────────────────────────────────────────────────────────┘

                              ↓
┌─────────────────────────────────────────────────────────────┐
│   On-going specialist palliative care intervention or         │
│                         discharge                             │
└─────────────────────────────────────────────────────────────┘
```

Figure 5.3   Referral pathway for specialist palliative care services

- Develop a monitoring role with a patient or with a site specific group of professionals.

Like all teams their achievements vary according to their structure, composition and the setting in which they work. Their role is largely an advisory one with many making a substantive educational contribution within the hospital. This has evolved partly because of their small number as well as the need to enable and facilitate others to provide their own effective palliative care.

Integrated Care Pathways (ICPs)

Integrated Care Pathways (ICPs) are an American import into the UK and involve the use of documentary tools used in a wide range of health care settings. In the current climate of clinical governance, ICPs are an example of tangible measures being used to demonstrate clinical effectiveness. Their use in palliative care enables practitioners to implement a structure for the effective organisation of nursing care for dying patients. They originated from the need to improve standards of patient care and were adopted for the care of the dying in all areas. ICPs enable professionals to highlight particular interventions which are appropriate once certain criteria are met. ICPs enable a holistic approach to be taken when carrying out the on-going assessment of patients' and relatives' needs. Much of the early work on ICPs for dying patients has been carried out by palliative care specialists, in particular, the Liverpool Care Pathway for the dying patient project. This project, which received NHS beacon status for its innovative patient centred care approach, is based on collaboration between Liverpool University hospitals and the Marie Curie Centre in Liverpool. Jointly, these centres have developed an integrated multi-professional care pathway as a means of developing and implementing a high standard of quality management for dying patients and their relatives. Riley (1998) points out that:

> ICPs determine locally agreed, multi-disciplinary practice based on guidelines and evidence, where available, for a specific patient/client group. It forms all or part of the clinical record, documents the care given and facilitates the evaluation of outcomes for continuous quality improvement.

ICPs are a good example of the type of care provided in hospices as well as many acute hospital settings. It should be made clear that ICPs, are not a standard item used in all contexts. Their emergence in the last decade has generated tremendous interest within the UK in a range of health care contexts and led to the introduction of a National Pathways Association. Currie (1998) reports on the results from an RCN survey pointing out that over 250 organisations are currently utilising ICPs in various forms. Their current use in palliative care contexts suggests that, within certain criteria, such as education and resource provision, they can be adopted by all health care professionals as a way of improving the care of patients receiving palliative care. In many ways they may be seen as a way of introducing palliative care principles within wider health care settings as Ellershaw et al (1997) point out:

> Care pathways are potentially appropriate for developing, monitoring and improving health care in the hospice, hospital and community.

The Liverpool Care Pathway (LCP) for the dying patient was adopted to transfer the hospice model of care into other care settings. The evidence suggests that nurses have generally found that the LCP model is capable of producing beneficial effects on patients and their families and is appreciated by doctors and nurses in hospitals (Jack et al 2003).

The purpose of Integrated Care Pathways

ICPs focus attention on the provision of the practical nursing care organised into a daily single record of nursing/health care with built in sections depending on the specific disease process. An ICP for a particular patient such as a terminally ill patient dying from cancer, is developed by a multi-disciplinary team (that can involve the patient and the family). Input into the plan can be derived from a range of sources such as research evidence, local policy and protocols and advice from medical experts. The ICP identifies a patient's actual and potential progress and acts as a check list for documenting when interventions are carried out by clinicians and other practitioners. This exists as a record for identifying whether there has been any deviation from the agreed plan (this can be very useful for conducting an audit trail to uncover retrospective clinical/nursing problems). Within the ICP, local guidelines such as the need for a CPR/Do Not Resuscitate protocol, or the use of opiates are an integral part of the plan and can be ticked off and potentially enable the ICP to be used as a legal document. This allows local established protocols to become more credible as well as facilitating the implementation of research into clinical practice. From this, it may be argued that ICPs are versatile tools interchangeable and valuable not only in terms of their potential for improving care but, more importantly in measuring and producing outcomes. Essentially they provide a method of assessing the impact of interventions using a cost base analysis whilst at the same time providing measures of quality that can be utilised to demonstrate the standards of care within a given context.

ICPs – the panacea of all ills?

It may be argued that ICPs cannot be introduced in all clinical areas especially where there is evidence of chronic under staffing due to long term sickness. There also needs to be a secure climate for change that is sustained by change agents or those who are able to promote a positive view of ICPs as well as monitoring their effectiveness. Should these issues not be identified and dealt with, then the introduction of ICPs could prove to be very difficult and counter-productive. ICPs represent a major and obvious beneficial source of care improvement and once formulated with a highly motivated team actually assist with the problems caused by sickness such as stress and poor morale. Ellershaw & Wilkinson (2003) point out that one of the key features of ICPs for the dying is that they empower generic health care workers to deliver optimal care to the dying which, at the same time enables them to access appropriate specialist support. The authors argue that the perennial problem of 'having no time to care for the dying' in hospital can be overcome by using ICPs because they enable staff to identify and implement care priorities. ICPs however are not the panacea of all ills and there are a number of limitations that need to be considered before they may be considered for use in all contexts. It may be argued that Integrated Care

Pathways emerged from within the business culture of health care provision and have their roots in the finance driven North American health care system (Chassin 1996, Zander 1998). An important consideration to be made about the use of the pathway is the type of patient and the nature of their condition. Ellershaw et al (1997) point out that dying patients should always be included who have specific criteria such as those who are being cared for in bed, semi-comatose and those unable to take sips of fluid or tablets. In this type of situation it is likely that the patient may have between 0–5 days in which to live. As a resource tool, they have tremendous potential for improving care. However, despite the amount of increasing research, their use, in most clinical areas where terminal care takes place has yet to be fully established. Health care teams should therefore be selective in the adoption of ICPs, in general based on the need to assess their value in relation to wider resource issues as well as their applicability in all contexts.

The need for teamwork

One of the key issues relating to the introduction of innovations to improve palliative care in hospitals in general and to adopt ICPs in particular is the need for education, and teamwork (Overill 1998, Ellershaw & Wilkinson 2003). In personal discussion Overill pointed out that ICPs were perhaps not easy to initiate in all areas, as individual units required the necessary staffing resources to implement them and staff needed to work together as a team to optimise the effect. The introduction and maintenance of ICPs is also problematic because of the need for resources, as well as contextual issues. First, in order to successfully develop ICPs you require a high level of motivation and support from members of the multi-disciplinary team who need to act as an integrated and cohesive whole. There is however little evidence of such cohesion in UK hospitals at present which casts doubt on the effectiveness of such innovations, unless the issues constraining the development of multi-disciplinary team-working are addressed, such as power relations between professional groups (Porter 1991). This is particularly relevant in certain hospital areas where nurses tend to be seen as the handmaidens of other professional groups particularly medical staff. It is not so apparent in other contexts such as in-patient and day hospice units where the type of hierarchical relations described by Porter (1991) exist. In particular, within nursing homes and residential centres for older people where medical staff are scarce, nurses often develop their own strategies for managing the care of dying patients, relating more towards the needs of the family and the patient and relying less on the dominance of other professional groups. The outcome of this absence of power and authority is a reliance on the wishes of the family and a need to preserve the integrity of the context in which care takes place, rather than risk fragmenting the team which has responsibility for the delivery of nursing care.

Summary

This chapter has highlighted several ways in which hospital palliative care can be improved by introducing hospice principles and practices. One of the key differences between hospices and hospitals is that the former are designed for the dying, but hospitals are charged with the huge responsibility for managing all sickness within society. Modern NHS Trust Hospitals operate on a different level to hospices in terms of population, administration and ideology. Socially, politically and economically, hospital culture varies tremendously, although this does not mean that the positive aspects of hospice care should not and cannot be incorporated into hospital care. Most nurses are aware of the positive influence resulting from increased human and material resources. Attempts to improve palliative care in hospitals by introducing specialist teams as well as managing and monitoring care using ICPs have made a positive impact, because they have enabled doctors and nurses who are able to work more closely together to monitor and improve patient progress.

Integrated Care Pathways are more likely to benefit areas that are receptive to change as well as able to use documentary tools effectively. In other words hospital wards with staffing problems and poor skill mix are unlikely to be able to utilise such approaches until the fundamental structural issues are addressed. In a similar way HBSPCTs are few in number and hospitals are very large and complex organisations. Ward staff may offer resistance to change and feel as if their care structures are being threatened by the so called experts. In some cases innovations such as ICPs and HBSPCTs may develop a life of their own, focusing importance on documenting care rather than providing practical care. The imposition of such change without an accurate assessment of its impact on the structures already in place is likely to have a negative outcome.

A well known and often debated issue relating to palliative care is the need to develop more effective forms of communication between all members of the multi-disciplinary team. Communication or a lack of, has been responsible for many problems within nursing today. Simply asking staff to work together as a team does not have the desired effect. Nurses and doctors should be able to spend time out of their normal routine and look at their communication, their strengths and weaknesses and focus on how to achieve more effective working practices for the benefit of patients and staff. To address team-working, it is important to consider allocating time and resources to allow teams to consider future aims and how to identify constraining issues. In hospitals, one of the problems is the issue of power between doctors and nurses. Power sharing and the creation of more egalitarian strategies of working are excellent ideals, although in practice may be problematic within certain contexts. However, by agreeing to consider issues such as this, hospital staff may become empowered to work more effectively as a team and for the benefit of the patient.

Reflecting on Part II, I conclude that initiating and sustaining change in hospitals is to some extent problematic. Many innovations within the NHS structure require time and resources as well as a commitment on the part of the organisation to embrace a sense of change. Moreover, the doctors and nurses involved may often perceive further change as reminders of the need to improve and work harder to meet increasingly more difficult goals.

Further reading

Ellershaw J. & Wilkinson S. (2003) *Care of the dying: a pathway to excellence.* Oxford University Press, Oxford.

This is a very interesting and well-written book with a foreword written by Cecily Saunders and a total of 17 contributors and nine chapters. The book looks back at the historical issues facing terminal care providers and also considers how ICPs may be used in places such as nursing homes.

The chapters focus on the use of Integrated Care Pathways and include a range of topics some of which adopt a 'how to approach' format and clearly describe what a pathway is. The chapters also deal with issues such as spirituality in the care of dying patients. The value of this book is that it provides more than a guide to introducing ICPs since it also considers the problems of caring for dying patients and the challenges facing palliative care providers.

Lawton J. (2000) *The dying process: patients' experiences of palliative care.* Routledge, London.

This book based on the author's doctoral research in a modern hospice provides an ethnographic account of the experiences of patients receiving palliative care. The author focuses on a revision of the concept of self and uses her study to provide a depiction of the process of dying. Some readers may find the book an uncomfortable read (especially those involved in hospice care). Some of my hospice colleagues have pointed out that the text does not flatter the providers of palliative care, mainly because it takes the notion of the body (somology) as its main focus and discusses the symbolic ways in which the patient as a body is dealt with and the inter-subjectivity between the patient, family and nurses. In doing so the book describes and critically analyses the processes involved in nursing care as the patient approaches death. The book is written in an academic style, but is very readable and above all, thought provoking for nurses and others involved in the care of dying patients in either a hospital or hospice setting.

McNamara B. (2001) *Fragile lives: death dying and care.* Open University Press, Buckingham.

This is an extremely well-written book about death and dying, based on the author's research using a sociological perspective. McNamara discusses a range of important issues including the medicalisation of death and the different cultural attitudes towards death, which affect us all. Written in an academic style, the text is readable and invigorating mainly because it is based on authentic accounts taken from research participants.

Part III
Caring in nursing home–residential home contexts

Part III focuses attention onto the care of dying patients in nursing and residential home settings. Chapter 6 examines the care dying patients receive in a nursing home setting. Chapter 7 considers terminal care in a residential care setting. Contextual differences will be discussed in terms of examining the way institutional care has certain similarities such as 'routines and house rules'. These two chapters consider the impact that death has on the family as well as the staff and other residents. One of the key features highlighted will be those practical issues associated with managing terminal care, when medical services are not readily available.

6

Life and death in a nursing home

Introduction

England has over 5,500 nursing homes providing long term care for 70,935 patients aged 65 and over, supported by their Local Authorities and more than 175,000 clients in residential care (Department of Health 2002). A significant number of people die each year in nursing homes, with figures indicating that 10% of all deaths in England take place in this context (Froggatt 2001).

The purpose of this chapter is to examine the long term care provided for older people in nursing home environments, in particular, the culture of care that exists in nursing home settings. To focus ideas around the care given in these types of establishments, I will give an account of my observations at Cedar House a residential/nursing home in the North West of England. I draw on accounts of the daily management of patients, giving an overview of the routine and features of this type of institutional care. Residents' and care staff perspectives supplement the account. Interviews with nurses and care assistants develop the descriptive features of the home, with short case studies of residents providing individual insights of the 'user's perspective'. The chapter also briefly reviews the move towards adopting palliative care principles in nursing homes and contrasts these with others described in previous chapters.

Cedar House

Cedar House is a 36-bedded mixed gender residential/nursing home situated in the North West of England. Some residents required nursing care, i.e. the attention of a registered nurse and others required social care from unqualified care staff. At the time of my visits the bed occupancy fluctuated between 94–100% and the ratio of men to women fluctuated around 1:8. Most of the referrals to Cedar House came from the local hospital trust social work team. Prior to admission the Registered Nurses at Cedar House (Jenny the Manager, and Carole her deputy) would carry out assessments of prospective residents. Few people came to Cedar House directly from home, although a few 'regular respite' clients, (those who were admitted to enable their carers to have a break), came from their own homes. This was achieved on an 'availability basis' since there were no designated respite beds at Cedar House which used to be a maternity hospital, orthopaedic unit and elderly care facility before it was sold to its current owners. The building itself was designed on two floors. Each floor had a lounge/dining room with residents' rooms adjacent and toilets and bathrooms close by. Most residents had their own rooms with five double rooms but no en-suite facilities. Invariably, residents tended to remain in the lounge of their own floor during the day, having their meals in the dining area and seldom venturing to the other floor. Each lounge had radio and tv/video facilities although these were not often in use during the day. Most Wednesdays there was entertainment in the downstairs lounge which many residents attended. Smoking was not permitted in the lounges, although there were outside areas for smokers. As you might expect residents tended to sit in the same places in the lounges where small social networks developed. Hairdressers, and a range of 'outsiders' including members of the church regularly visited the home as well as relatives and visitors. My first impression was very positive. The lounges were 'socially noisy', with much chatter and talking going on and staff having a background presence.

The staff

The staff consisted of two registered nurses, and 12 care assistants. The day shift consisted of one nurse and three care assistants on each of the two floors. There was no internal rotation of staff between day and night duty. The night shift consisted of one registered nurse and three care assistants. To cover the home the staff operated a three shift system with 'earlies' (starting at 07.15) and 'lates' (12.30–20.45). The care assistants undertook 12 hour shifts in order to make up the required number of hours in their contract. Cedar House had four level three (NVQ) care staff. Agency nurses (often the same ones) were also used to supplement the shifts and to cover when the regular staff were on sick leave. The staff at the home were supported by two full-time cooks, (one working 8–6 Monday to Friday and the other covering the weekend) two kitchen assistants and two domestics.

Cedar House operated a key worker system which involved each resident having a care assistant designated to ensure that their individual needs were met. This involved a range of duties from ensuring they had sufficient personal clothing for example toiletries and new stockings, to liaising with relatives and outside agencies about their day to day living. The key worker system had a number of organisational functions in terms of making sure that the resident's individual needs were met by ensuring that the designated key worker reported any particular care needs to the registered nurse and paid special attention to their particular resident. In conjunction with the home administrator, the nurses dealt with financial affairs. The home administrator also acted as accountant and receptionist together with a host of other roles. The day to day routine was fairly flexible with breakfast being available almost anytime up until 11.00 hours. Lunch was served at 12.30 and was the biggest meal of the day. The evening meal or 'tea' was at 16.30 hours.

Residents

Staff at Cedar House described their admission system as an 'open door policy' which meant that they invariably admitted patients with a range of problems. The Cedar House resident population tended to come from hospitals and in many ways were familiar with institutional patterns of care where the staff and routine dominated their daily lives. Table 6.1 provides an overview of the admission criteria at Cedar House. Few residents were discharged to their own home and the majority stayed at Cedar House until they died, which meant that few beds became available for another admission. The resident population therefore tended to be rather static. In other circumstances, residents with mental health problems may be admitted and then transferred to another home or

Table 6.1 Inclusion and exclusion criteria for admission to Cedar House

Inclusion criteria	Exclusion criteria
People with social/welfare needs who require 24-hr care	Patients with serious mental health problems (psychosis)
Those with no primary carer in the home	Those with aggressive/violent behaviour
Patients with specific nursing problems such as leg ulcers	Patients with advanced dementia (those at high risk)
Those requiring nursing care	Patients requiring specialist care

mental health establishment for further treatment or long term care. Some of the residents of Cedar House received nursing care for a variety of problems associated with their inability to carry out Activities of Daily Living (ADL), such as washing, dressing and mobility. Others had specific health problems such as a chronic leg ulcer requiring the intervention of a nurse. Other residents required social care and made up approximately 30% of the residents at Cedar House. The status of residents changed according to their need and if a 'residential client' required nursing care, they would be assessed by a social worker and a case made to 'rebadge' their status, which meant that the patient could receive nursing care from the nurses which they were technically ineligible for unless they had been assessed. The categorisation of residents in this way is important since technically if a residential client requires medical/nursing care, for example as a result of an acute problem, the staff are required to call an ambulance to take them to hospital (if the circumstances warrant this). A recent episode supported this where a resident had an asthma attack, from which she recovered, but later the GP asked if the nurses could look after her. The resident was in receipt of residential care and unfortunately, because of the protocols, had to be taken to hospital. In practice, nurses felt obliged in certain cases to treat 'non-nursing' residents, as an exception to the rule, provided that they were re-categorised as nursing residents in the future. A key issue here is that nursing residents, because of the cost, have to pay increased fees. The home is also strictly controlled in terms of changes in the ratio of nursing residents to registered nurses. Alterations in numbers requiring nursing care mean that more nurses have to be employed. The general assessment of patients was on-going and using a key worker system as well as nursing assessment, the needs of residents were monitored and reviewed regularly. The general philosophy of Cedar House was based on the belief that the home was the resident's home and the aim of the care provided was to enable the residents to live a good quality of life until they eventually died. This included ensuring that their needs were met at all levels including physical, psychological and social. The staff made efforts to organise outside visits including pubs and shopping trips.

An important aspect of life at Cedar House was visiting which took place most of the day, although few outsiders visited in the morning. There were regular groups of visitors who came every day although most people visited their relatives at the weekend and in the evening.

Institutional care

One of the striking things about Cedar House, in contrast to other areas I visited, was the relaxed but stimulating atmosphere when you entered. The downstairs lounge with its numerous chairs reflected the fact that it was an establishment for older people, but the first impression was of a lively household much different to NHS establishments. I wondered how different it felt to staff at Cedar House who had previous experiences of NHS care. According to Carole in response to the question 'How different is life at Cedar House to life in the NHS?'

> Completely different, you can't even begin to compare it the fact is people live here it's their home, for example residents who want a cup of tea want it now, it's no use to them saying you can't have it now. They expect you (quite rightly) to go an' get it then.

Sally, pointed out that:

> The staff know the residents much more than you would in the NHS, they know what they like and what they don't like.

A care assistant explained the general philosophy of Cedar House in terms of a comparison between NHS and residential/nursing home care catering:

> Residents are given choices, there is a three week menu that 'rolls over', if a patient doesn't like a certain meal then we get them another one, basically they don't have to eat what is on offer at the time. That's one of the key differences.

The staff at Cedar House identified a number of key differences between their perceptions of NHS care and life at Cedar House. These included the flexibility of the staff to cater for individual needs, the extent to which residents received individual attention and the degree to which everyday activity remained at an informal level. An example of this was the cook who provided food for individual residents who did not like the particular meal on the menu or required a specific type of food. The staff pointed out that it is in their interests, and that of the resident, that individual client needs are met. On a number of occasions, care staff pointed out that residents are more highly thought of than hospital patients. Cedar House was their home and they will invariably spend the rest of their lives there.

Staff and residents

One of the key issues associated with the quality of care in any institutional setting is the atmosphere created by those who live and work there. This largely stemmed from the type of interpersonal relations predominate in the home. In relation to the care of patients in a nursing home setting, Ford & Heath (1996) point out that older people value the positive contact and meaningful engagement that is offered by the staff. In Cedar House, I observed a range of relationships being developed and maintained between the staff and the residents. At the heart of any client/resident staff relationship is the caring attitude of the staff member whether they are care assistants, kitchen staff or the matron/manager. Clearly staff attitudes emanate from good leadership and high standard role models. The home manager is therefore the key to enabling and facilitating good relationships at all levels in the home since it is the manager who ultimately takes responsibility for ensuring the overall quality of the care. The home manager's role is multifaceted. He/she has the management responsibility for ensuring that standards of care remain high, staff and resident morale is maintained and that a healthy balance is maintained between the owner's need for financial constraints and the requirement to provide an effective high quality of care for all residents. Ford & Heath (1996:51) assert that:

> Nurses should have a close interpersonal relationship with their clients (in order to be) effective in contributing to their life satisfaction.

The focus placed on nurses and their caring role needs to extend to all care staff, since the evidence from my research in residential and nursing home settings suggests that the care assistants in both settings provided the majority of the individual and personal care to the residents. A number of writers have attempted to define care in terms of it being associated with kindness and a sense of nurturing the individual (Smith 1992). However, for many 'true caring' consists of a range of attributes that include carrying out tasks efficiently, and attending to the psychosocial and emotional needs of the client (Griffin 1981). In discussion with residents at Cedar House, I felt that what many were saying to me about their perceptions of caring was not based on the explicit 'high profile' type of care which involved administration, such as arranging for their hospital appointments and doctors visits. Whilst important care considerations, many pointed out that it was the small detail, such as having patience when they were not able to use the toilet quickly or the acts of kindness in making sure that the carer went back to their room for their favourite soap. The following comments are responses to the question 'what type of things do you appreciate the staff doing for you that you consider to be caring?'

- I appreciate it when the staff look out for me and allow me to catch their eye when I need something and there is no one about.
- I like it when they ask me is there anything else they can do for me.

- I am a pain at times and I'm sure they get fed up with me so I particularly like it when someone smiles at me and makes me feel better inside.

Residents' perceptions focused around the unspoken gestures and the attention paid by the carer to small detail such as anticipating that a resident prefers to sit within a particular group of residents and away from the radio. Therefore, in response to the question *what do residents value in care staff?*, it appears that many appreciate the small acts of human kindness that may often go unnoticed but are much appreciated and demonstrate a form of moderated love towards those one has a duty to provide care to.

Terminal care: death at Cedar House

Cedar House did not have a specific remit to admit terminally ill patients as some nursing homes do. Where this applies, the National Association of Health Authorites and Trusts (1991) have produced guidelines to support and educate staff about their specific duties towards the patient and their families. The care of residents who are dying is an important part of life in most nursing homes and many of the nurses and care staff have an abundance of experience in caring for terminally ill residents. The Care Standards Act (Department of Health 2000a), which defines national minimum standards for care homes, states that:

> Palliative care, practical assistance and advice and bereavement counselling are provided by professional/specialist agencies if the service user wishes.

The *National Service Framework (NSF) for Older People* (Department of Health 2001) in its report acknowledges that older people approaching the end of life may have a need for palliative care. The report recommends that information giving, the management of symptoms (including pain), psychosocial care and bereavement support are provided to older people and their relatives in order to ensure that at the appropriate time, their end of life experiences are managed professionally. An important consideration here is that care staff maximise privacy, dignity and elements such as spiritual care.

In common with many institutions for older people, the number of deaths in Cedar House varied, with some residents only staying a few weeks before they died and others who remained in the home for many years. On average there were 12–15 deaths per year, mostly expected, although occasionally some were sudden. Where a patient dies suddenly and they have not been seen by a doctor (GP) in the last 14 days there is a post mortem and the GP is unable to sign a death certificate until the coroner has investigated the death. In other circumstances, residents who became ill, were seen by the GP and if they did not require hospitalisation were cared for in the home, invariably in their own bedroom under the supervision of the nurses:

> We tend to nurse people in their own rooms for greater privacy and personal comfort.

This was said to enable the resident to have more privacy although others would argue that this helps to separate the (dying) resident from the living and is of more practical benefit to the staff (Miller 1985). Residents who became ill and required specific nursing care such as intravenous and blood transfusions would not be cared for in the home, although the nursing staff managed certain forms of feeding such as PEG infusion lines.

Care at the end of life

When a resident is dying, the staff at Cedar House try to accommodate the needs of the resident and the family at all times. This can include facilitating visitors to visit at any time, including friends, members of the clergy and other residents who may wish to visit the dying resident in their room. Requests for any type of service such as the use of music to be played or for the resident to visit a particular place were accommodated as well as respecting residents' wishes to be left alone. The aim of care at this time was to enable the resident to have, what many refer to as, a 'good death'.

On one occasion, the home received an unusual request to admit a hospice patient for terminal care. Some would argue that this is likely to become a more frequent occurrence (Froggatt 2000). The patient had been in a local hospice but did not want to die there and requested to die at home. Because he could not be cared for in his own home, he asked to be admitted to Cedar House to spend the last few weeks of life there. His request was to die 'in his home town' so he was transferred to Cedar House and died after a few weeks. There were no specific policies for terminal care at Cedar House, no Integrated Care Pathways, or special documentation. The staff appeared to have a broad aim of ensuring that the resident and the family's wishes were met as far as the resources of the home allowed. This included ensuring that all physical care was of a high quality with limited intervention unless it was necessary, such as not insisting that the resident has a bath or even be assisted in washing unless they requested so. During times of staff/resident contact psychological care was maintained through the intervention of key workers and nurses who focused attention on the resident's needs and liaised with the GP if the patient required medical attention.

The death of a resident

The death of a resident at Cedar House was seen as an important but sad event although it was not given such a high profile in terms of the lack of rituals expressed in some areas, partly because it was seen as an inevitable aspect of the resident's life. Clearly, as residents are reminded when they are admitted, death is a natural outcome and one which needs to be prepared for. When a resident is admitted, they or their family are asked if they have given any thought to whether the resident has a preference for cremation or burial or do they have any special preferences about the funeral arrangements? Asking the resident/family this question when the resident is in good health serves two purposes. The first is practical in the sense that it enables the staff to provide the necessary information to the funeral directors when the patient dies. Secondly, in a symbolic sense it can serve as a reminder in some cases of the reality that the resident is, in the future likely to die during their time at Cedar House. This can take some relatives back when asked, as Jenny, the Manager points out:

> When you ask about cremation or burial most relatives look at you as if to say what do you mean? It's a funny thing to ask when a resident is first admitted.

A number of writers commenting on the care provided to older people in nursing homes at the end of life, have been critical of the quality of care. Frogatt et al (2001) point out that confusion about who is responsible for providing nursing care (especially for residential settings), may lead to inconsistencies in care. Counsel and Care (1995) in their research study based on the management of death and dying in six residential and nursing homes, point out that in some cases the key problem identified with the death of a resident was poor communication, although they also cite examples of 'good deaths'. The report describes a situation when a resident died and the nurse went to make 'the necessary arrangements'. Whilst doing so the deceased resident's daughter arrived in the home, went past reception and found her mother who looked asleep, but, as the daughter discovered, had died peacefully minutes earlier. It may be useful to reflect in more detail on this authentic account taken from the Counsel and Care research.

However, under the direction of the NHS Cancer Plan (Department of Heath 2000), which seeks to provide palliative care education for community nurses, it is envisaged that this type of care for patients in nursing and residential care settings would become more widely available in the future.

Management of the deceased

When a resident died, the nurse in charge was required by protocol to initially inform the General Practitioner of the death who would then have to confirm death. Legally, the nurses had no right to confirm death until a medical practitioner had seen the resident. This can lead to problems in terms of the timing of when to inform the relatives.

Once the GP has confirmed death, the relatives and next of kin were informed and arrangements were made with the funeral director of their choice to come to the home and pick up the deceased resident. In most cases, residents used one of two local funeral directors. Since both knew the individual layout of the home, discretion was used in entering and leaving the home so as to avoid any unnecessary embarrassment to other residents. In some cases a stretcher trolley was used to carry the deceased, in other cases, a body bag was used, largely depending on the size and weight of the resident.

It may be useful to provide some kind of practical marker to indicate when a patient has died. In one nursing home, the staff would light a candle in the foyer entrance when a patient died to indicate to other residents and visitors that a resident had died. This stimulated questions as to who has died and also enabled others to acknowledge the death publicly by making a contribution for flowers or pay their respects to grieving family members. In some cases, the death of a resident could be seen as a source of relief in the sense that if the resident was distressed or in pain before they died others may consider it a blessing that the *end had come*.

Caring for a dying resident: Edna

Edna was a 91 year old lady who developed broncho-pneumonia in December. Although Edna had Alzheimer's disease she was often quite cheerful and despite being cared for in bed the staff would ensure that she came into the lounge and spend time with the other residents as she had periods when she seemed quite lucid. When she became tired and unable to manage being out of bed, the staff would take her back to her room and make her comfortable. An important part of caring for residents who were ill and becoming terminal was ensuring that they had as much social contact as they could. This seemed to be important to the staff at Cedar House. Perhaps it was to do with not hiding the fact of death away from others. Clearly there were practical issues in bringing residents into the lounge, for example the staff could observe them and make sure that they did not die suddenly and alone. Sue, the Care Assistant recalls how her mother had died in a nursing home and at times she recalls how lonely her mother must have felt being in bed isolated. Brykczynska (1992:9) points out that having empathy for a patient need not depend on personal experience but 'rather on our level of sensitivity and common human understanding of life and life's events'. Sometimes our personal experience influences the way we behave although this does not mean that those who have little experience (of stressful life events) cannot provide high quality sensitive care. Providing good leadership can shape quality care at the end of life as well as adequate resources and a determination to facilitate the kind of experiences we might want to have if we, or our loved ones were in the client's position.

Residents' accounts of life in nursing homes

Often listening to residents and also learning about their perceptions can help us to make sense of what we as professional carers should be aiming for. Ellen Newton, a freelance writer, provides a powerful and very moving account of life in a nursing home, based on the diary she made of her experiences. This eventually became a book which chronicled the six years she spent in a series of nursing homes. At the age of 81, she had had enough and decided to discharge herself from hospital and with the help of her family found a small flat and began making her living writing about her experiences as an inmate in many nursing homes. The following are extracts from her book *This bed my centre* Newton (1980:81):

> June Monday: Day begins here at 5.00 am. No early morning cup of tea. Breakfast at 7.30. The main meal is at midday. There is afternoon tea poured into your cup as your nursing aid of tea at the moment likes it.
>
> [p147] This June has dragged its slow length along. This morning at six the temperature was only 1 degree C. much bed. Pain. And distress over things that I cannot alter, things that common sense tells me to accept, and simply not let myself be disturbed by. It's a strange segregation. There are never less than three or four who are mentally very sick people. Their much heard voices are sometimes like shrill brawling, sometimes like off-key, sounding brass – to say nothing of the odd ones who, day or night may wander pointlessly in and out of my room. They all need care and compassion. They may need it far more than I do. But there should be a special place and special skills to provide it for them.

My observations at Cedar House and conversations with residents and staff led me to believe that it was a nice place to be and that the staff tried hard to ensure that they did the best they could for the residents. It was made clear to me that whilst the staff often pointed out that it was the residents' home, many residents would have preferred to have lived in their own home and regarded Cedar House as second best.

The following accounts from residents in the home include a 'proxy account' from one relative and provide a mixed snap-shot view of how individuals came to be at Cedar House and how they managed their day to day activity.

Edgar

Edgar was a 90 year old widower who had been at Cedar House as a nursing resident for 5 years. He was admitted as a result of a stroke which made it difficult for him to dress and wash himself at home. Edgar and his wife Jean, an insulin dependent diabetic, were admitted as a couple and shared a downstairs room until Jean had both legs amputated and then, after suffering a stroke, died in hospital. That was two years ago and the memory of her death still makes Edgar very upset. Edgar lived next to the office on the ground floor and was clearly seen as a 'good resident' in that he was always polite, an able communicator, and invariably cheerful. He woke early (at 06.30) as he enjoyed a smoke and spent the first few minutes of the day outside by the back door. He was partially sighted and although he could hear the television he rarely watched it except for the football. Edgar felt that it was important that his room was close to the toilet as he needed to go in the night and usually managed without assistance.

> I like to be my own boss, I like being independent and not having to rely on the staff all the time. Oh they are a great lot but they are kept busy with some of them here.

Edgar rarely went upstairs to join other residents and preferred to stay in the downstairs lounge. He had only spent one day upstairs when the downstairs lounge was decorated. He enjoyed the food, and in particular, he liked the fact that it was quiet downstairs at night. Edgar is very happy at Cedar House and seemed content to spend the rest of his life there.

Betty

Betty was an 87 year old lady who lived in the upstairs of Cedar House and was very bright and cheerful despite being occasionally quite confused as a result of Alzheimer's disease. Betty gave a rather mixed account of her life, pointing out that she considered herself fortunate to be independent in terms of her mobility. She was admitted to the home following an operation on her bladder and her husband was unable to cope with her at home when she was discharged partly because of the Alzheimer's and also because he was advancing in years himself. Betty explained that she felt lucky because she was able to mobilise around the home (upstairs) whenever she wanted. She explained how it was different for those (residents) who relied on the staff to get them about:

> I'm alright, I use my stick and get about on my own going to the toilet and up to the table, it's those who have to wait I feel sorry for at times.

Despite her confusion, Betty was able to explain how when the staff are busy some residents who are dependent on help to mobilise are unable to do what they want because of the need to wait until staff are free to lift them or help them get up.

Emma

Emma was a 93 year old lady who was admitted to Cedar House after showing signs of dementia for many years and being unable to care for herself at home. Her gradual deterioration, forgetfulness and constant lack of thought when it came to shutting doors, turning off the gas and wandering around not knowing why she was going outside in the early hours of the night, caused her family and herself distress and necessitated admission. The home agreed that she could bring her pet cat Tommy with her which made the transition much easier and he became a Cedar House pet. Emma remained confused and unsteady on her feet and things came to a head when she fell down stairs and fractured her femur. This necessitated a stay in hospital and after a fairly traumatic time on the orthopaedic ward of the local hospital, Emma returned to the home having survived the operation. Her mental state had deteriorated but she managed with her limited mobility. Her three children visited and noticed the gradual changes in her overall condition. Emma is dependent on the staff in terms of her mobility and washing and dressing. The main concern of the staff is her mobility as she still continues to want to get up and walk around unaided. One care assistant pointed out:

> Emma, is a bit of a worry at times as she wants to get up but we can't always allow her to wander in case she falls, and hurts herself or another resident.

Residents who are at risk from falls such as Emma, pose problems when the home is very busy and under staffed. In general people like Emma who are confused and like to wander, are looked after by the staff who tend to sit with them or take them into the office if they have written work to do.

The relatives' perspective

Thomas's mother was a resident at Cedar House. She had been there for five years and he was pleased with the care she received, although at times he worried about whether she received sufficient attention.

> It's a general concern I think, it's not that she isn't well cared for, it's perhaps that I can't always be there and know what she wants because she cannot tell me.

When his mother was first admitted (with a CVA) he worried about her a lot perhaps because of the media stories of neglect and also because of the wide variety of care available since the proliferation of private nursing homes. To a certain extent, relatives carry with them a degree of sustained uncertainty about whether their loved ones are receiving the care they need. Some relatives who lived close to Cedar House visited every day:

> Yes we come every day and see Nan, it's not far and we are retired, so it's not so bad and she likes to see us.

Other relatives who do not live close by, visit regularly but are unable to be aware of the day to day activities and rely on staff to keep them informed. This is an important part of the role of the staff who relatives rely on for information.

Palliative care and nursing homes

Nursing homes are now required to provide care for a frail population of people without the essential resources (Maddocks 1996). The increasing numbers of people discharged from hospital and the increased number of beds in nursing homes suggests that nursing homes are key areas when it comes to the provision of palliative care. Palliative care is a term that has been in use since the late 1980s (1987 was the first time palliative medicine was recognised as a medical specialty). Before this time people often referred to patients with life threatening conditions from which they were likely to die as needing terminal care. Since this time, palliative medicine and nursing care has proliferated considerably with a wide range of opinions about the appropriateness of this type of approach. In some cases palliative care is seen as being synonymous with the kind of terminal care provided to the dying person. In other places such as the larger hospices, palliative care co-exists with what some would argue to be acute medical intervention such as blood transfusions, cardiac monitoring and even cardiopulmonary resuscitation (Costello & Horne 2003). Terminal care is generally considered to be an intrinsic part of the palliative nursing care and medical treatment provided to a patient whose death is considered to be imminent within a matter of days, weeks or months. Field (1998:111) points out that whilst palliative care contains the idea that death is likely to happen, it is often concerned with the alleviation of symptoms and the enhancement of the patient's quality of life. Consistent with all aspects of palliation, the care provided extends to the patient and the family. The latter in some cases becomes the focus of the practitioner's attention when for example the patient's condition is stabilised and the emotional needs of the family become a priority. One of the contemporary aims of the palliative care movement in Britain is to diversify and promote its aims within a wider context. Froggatt (2000) points out that nursing home staff are encouraged to adopt a palliative care approach when caring for older people at the end of life, although it is not always easy to apply palliative care principles within a nursing home setting (Maddocks 1996). There are a number of reasons for this, including confusion about the roles and responsibilities of care staff and nurses, in particular where residents are not classified as 'nursing residents' and the community nursing services are required to manage an acute problem, such as a leg ulcer when there are nurses in the home. This situation highlighted by Froggatt et al (2001) is made more complex when the resident is dying and in need of intervention from community nurses.

There is also a need to address the fundamental issue of what may be regarded as palliative care and terminal care. For most of the staff at Cedar House, the latter applied to those residents who were clearly very ill and dying. It tended to extend towards the need for carrying out physical care more than attending to the psychosocial needs of the resident. The more complex areas of care such as emotional involvement and the provision of spiritual care may require greater education provision that many homes currently receive.

The research evidence suggests that care assistants play a key role in the palliative care of residents who are dying (Miskella & Avis 1998). It is also clear that like others, the values and attitudes of care assistants has an impact on the overall quality of care and the way in which residents perceived their ability to care for them. The comments I received from nurses at the home suggested that much of the 'nursing and care work' was carried out by care assistants, a finding similar to that in hospitals where nursing auxiliaries and student nurses were found to have the most contact with patients. There is also a growing need to 'open up' nursing home care so as to involve other nurses and specialist practitioners. By working collaboratively nursing home staff and specialist practitioners can help to establish and develop the highest possible level of palliative care. This can be achieved by effective education and training.

Summary

The projected increase in the older population together with the movement of long term care from the NHS indicate that nursing homes will play a key role in the provision of terminal care for older people. This chapter has raised many issues associated with the care of dying older people. The nursing home context with the emphasis on it being the resident's home has great potential for reflecting the type of death experiences not seen in hospitals or hospices. This does not however prevent certain features of the institutional care of dying residents being expressed which reflect the institution's needs being met before those of the resident. Cedar House seemed to have adopted a set of flexible rules and routines determined much more by the need for individual care. This may explain the more intimate nature of these institutions and be influenced by the small number of residents and the greater involvement of relatives in end of life decision making.

One of the key issues in caring for the dying in non-hospital contexts is the lack of available medical services. Despite this, many nurses and care workers appeared to manage the end of life issues by developing their social structures to anticipate and prepare for death. The overarching feature of the management of death and dying in each context demonstrates the way in which the nursing and social care is constructed through the interactions of the carers. In turn these subjective experiences of death help to shape the social structures that prevail and sustain the culture for dealing with dying patients. The examination of non-hospital settings continues in the next chapter with an account of life and death in a residential care setting.

Further reading

Garrett G. (1994) *Healthy ageing.* Wolfe Publishing, London.

This collection of 45 formerly published papers written by both nurse practitioners and academics makes an excellent contribution to knowledge and awareness of the experiences of older people. The range of topics from nutrition and pain to family care provide a sound and very readable account of the challenges faced by nurses caring for older people.

Katz J., Komaromy C. & Sidell M. (1995) *Death and dying in residential and nursing homes for older people – examining the case for palliative care.* Report for the Department of Health. London.

This report provides an account of the research project by the Open University, which examined the extent to which palliative care principles have become integrated into nursing home settings.

Lee E. (1995) *A good death: a guide for patients and carers facing terminal illness at home.* Rosendale Press, London.

Written by a GP this book designed for dying patients and their carers gives a clear and comprehensive account of the practical issues associated with terminal care at home. Although each individual's death is unique, some of the practical issues can be prepared for and anticipated. This book is an interesting and very practical guide that is well-written and aimed at those who make the difficult decision to care for their loved ones at home.

Newton E. (1980) *This bed my centre*. Virago, London.

This book is an account of one woman's experiences of living 6 years in a nursing home. Written as a diary the book provides a moving portrayal depicting scenarios of life in private nursing homes in Britain. The personal although objective writing gives the reader a personal insight into the sadness that was one person's experience.

Rose X. (1995) *Widows journey*. Souvenir Press, London.

This book is written by a widow and provides a very clear account of the experiences of a woman whose world famous husband (Leonard Rose) died of leukaemia. In many ways this book reads like a novel, although like many biographical accounts such as *A grief observed*, by C.S. Lewis, (1961) the author's accounts have tremendous sincerity and leave one feeling that the description of feelings resonate so well with the reader's personal experiences.

7

Living and dying in a residential care setting

Introduction

In the UK, deaths occurring outside hospital have become an important topic of debate (Maddocks & Parker 2001) and in contemporary times, almost 20% of deaths occur in nursing or residential care facilities (Field & Froggatt 2003). Death in residential care in the UK each year, despite the limited research, has an impact on both the staff and residents (Peace et al 1997). In 2001, the number of supported residents in Local Authority residential, independent residential, nursing, and un-staffed homes increased to 265,100. This represents an increase of 3,300 on the previous year (Department of Health 2002). Over half (56%) of supported residents were in independent residential care, 27% in independent nursing homes and 14% in Local Authority staffed homes. The vast majority of all supported residents (78%) were aged 65 or more.

In this chapter, I describe the care and daily management of residents in Newlands, a Local Authority residential care home for older people. The chapter describes the structural features of the home and the challenges facing both staff and residents who share their lives within a context in which there is a limited amount of active nursing care taking place compared to the social care being provided. In particular I draw on the concept of 'social death' (Sweeting & Gilhooley 1991) to develop an image of life that exists outside of mainstream society where residents adopt a routine existence that revolves around a range of activities largely social in nature. The death of a resident was relatively unusual and when this occurred, it was treated as a much less dramatic event than in other institutional settings. One of the central features of the chapter is the practical issues that together make up the pattern of activity that assists in the construction of what is being called 'social death', the lack of social interaction and meaningful engagement with the outside world which can occur in some institutional settings.

The chapter includes a description of two case studies. Martha, depicts the reluctance of one resident whose phrase '*I will be better off if I wasn't here*' is contrasted with the experience of another (Alice), who has little social contact with others due to advanced dementia and although physically able and not requiring nursing care, does require a tremendous amount of social care in order to maintain her precarious existence. The chapter will draw attention to the contextual differences between residential and other institutional settings and compare features of two different models of care (warehousing and horticultural) and the extent to which these predominate in residential care settings.

Newlands

Newlands, is a 17-bedded Local Authority residential home offering 24 hour personal care to older people within a catchment area that includes a population of 30,000. The building itself had a long tradition as a residential home, although originally it was the home of a wealthy local family. Over the years it has been modified to become a home with numerous adaptations enabling it to house a group of frail elderly people. The average age of the residents was 82 with few under the age of 75 and one older lady about to celebrate her 100th birthday. Two of the 17 beds were reserved for assessment and short term care. At the time of my visits the ratio of female to male residents was 13:2. In most cases residents had single rooms but there were three double rooms, two of which were designated as long stay. The home was also being upgraded in accordance with changes taking place in care home legislation (Department of Health 2002) to enable all residents to have a single room. During the day Newlands also took eight day care residents, brought to the home by a volunteer transport scheme. It was difficult to assess residents average length of stay, although it was clear that this was of several years duration. The physical geography consisted of a main hallway and lounge area together with two further lounges (one for smoking), each had TV and video. There was also a conservatory with easy chairs and a pay phone.

Admission to Newlands

The majority of residents arrived at Newlands via social work referral. The local hospitals provided many of the clients who, for 'social reasons' such as being unable to care for themselves, find themselves in the position of looking for temporary or in some cases a permanent place to live. Residents who seek a place at Newlands are required to be mentally alert and able to look after themselves as much as possible. As far as possible, on referral, residents need to have a reasonable level of independence, which often means that they are continent, mobile and able to look after themselves with the minimum of supervision. It is recognised however, that over time, their physical and mental condition deteriorates and they can become more dependent on care staff. Referrals are not made where residents are in need of nursing care or those who have severe problems with activities of daily living such as being incontinent. Most residents at Newlands however needed some form of assistance with personal care such as washing, dressing, bathing and using the toilet. Over the years residents were admitted with colostomies and a range of other prostheses. One of the difficult issues is the prospective residents' mental state. As far as possible, residents with advanced senile dementia were not referred. This was a problematic issue and a 'grey area', which I discussed with care staff. Carol (Deputy Manager) pointed out that:

> We don't like psychiatric patients that's for sure, our recent experience of residents with mental health issues has made us very wary. We don't have the training and find it very difficult to deal with some of the abuse you have to put up with. Dementia is ok, we are used to that and are quite good at handling residents with Alzheimer's.

I observed many residents with varying degrees of senile dementia, which the staff pointed out, developed during their stay at Newlands. It became clear that in the main, these residents were unproblematic to the staff and were also tolerated well by the vast majority of fellow residents. The most significant division of residents in Newlands was the one between male and female. The two male residents (both smokers) spent their time in the smoking lounge where they appeared to enjoy their separation from female residents who congregated as a group in the large lounge. This group consisted of those who were clearly suffering from dementia as well as those who were mentally alert. Like many institutional settings, Newlands had an institutional appearance despite the ornate and elaborate architecture. As a result of the many fire and health and safety regulations and the need to have fire proof furnishings, there were few material possessions in residents' rooms and often bags of personal clothes could not be stored. The preservation of personal dignity was a high priority for staff, who maintained this through observing 'rules' about entering a resident's room and ensuring that bathing and washing were private affairs. This was a pleasant contrast to my many years spent in hospital settings where patients seemed to shed their dignity at the same time as their clothes, for their first medical examination. The aims and objectives of Newlands were proudly displayed on the main notice board outside the office (see Figure 7.1).

Aims and Objectives

To provide a safe and friendly home for elderly residents, with good care standards making sure individuals' opinions are respected and met.
To improve the opportunity for residents to make choices.
To make sure continuity takes place within the home on care standards.
To meet the standards as set out in the minimum Care Standards Act 2002.
To continue to audit our work and to make sure client needs are met.
To facilitate community links by providing short term and daily care.
To promote rights of all residents in all respects of health and social life.

Figure 7.1   Newlands: aims and objectives

A day in the life of Newlands

The documented information about Newlands states that '... no set routine operates and residents may go to bed whenever they wish'. However, whilst residents did choose when they went to bed, a routine did exist largely because like many other care institutions, residents need to structure their lives and develop a sense of reality. A typical day at Newlands began with the staff arriving for the early shift and the handover from the night staff. Invariably this involved just the deputy manager. This took about 20 minutes and involved an exchange of information about the events in the night, who woke up, who went to the toilet and who did not sleep. Most of the residents at Newlands went to bed early and woke early, with the exception of those who watched TV until late in the evening. Breakfast in the dining room was usually well attended and residents invariably chose a cooked breakfast of eggs, or cereal and toast. Breakfast took place from 08.15 hours onwards. After breakfast, the TV was switched on and residents made their way to the lounge (via the toilets) with a number assisted by the staff. Some residents had their meals in the non-smoking lounge.

The morning period for residents was spent like the rest of the day in the lounge, newspapers were delivered, some residents got up later and others watched TV. The morning routine was punctuated by residents receiving the medication prescribed by their GPs and dispensed by the manager/deputy manager. The staff were invariably busy with two care workers and an assistant manager on duty making beds, tidying rooms and helping residents into the lounge. A number of residents required help with washing and dressing and this occupied the bulk of the early part of the morning. Those residents who developed problems such as leg ulcers requiring the services of the district nurse would be seen regularly in their rooms when the nurses visited. The district nurses seemed to enjoy a good relationship with the care staff and were willing to give advice on a range of nursing care and health related issues such as the effects of medication.

The role of home cook was an important and busy one (sometimes the role of the cook was taken up by the care staff if the cook was off sick). Cook prepared the most substantial meal of the day at lunchtime (12.15 hours onwards) which consisted of the resident's main three course meal and was taken in the dining room.

The afternoon was spent in a similar way to the morning with the majority of residents sat in the lounge. Visitors to Newlands invariably made an appearance during the afternoon and in the evening. The evening meal or 'tea' (16.15–16.45) was often a choice of sandwiches or snacks and was much lighter than the midday meal. I was unable to discern whether the rationale for the meals was based on the needs of the cook (who left at 16.30), and the organisation, or the individual needs of the residents. In the evening, supper was served at 20.30. Throughout the day, a variety of drinks were available (served by staff mid morning and afternoon) to residents and their guests on request, as well as being dispensed from a machine, although this was rarely used.

Social therapy

Music from the radio and TV was an integral part of the social milieu. Most care facilities encourage residents to engage in social therapy and Newlands was no exception. The classical game of bingo, board games, newspaper reading, quizzes and a range of discussions helped to stimulate staff and residents, particularly if the focus of the activity enabled residents to reflect on their own lives. Reminiscence therapy, whereby older people were encouraged to reflect back on their past lives and recall previous events, can be a very rewarding activity that also has proven therapeutic value. Sadly, my observations during the short time I spent at Newlands, did not include a great deal of social activity. The television and radio were the most consistent forms of stimulation that the majority of residents engaged with. In particular two male residents spent the majority of their time in the TV lounge which also doubled as a smoking room and this became their domain, with few others entering unless they wanted to smoke. There were however a number of outside services such as chiropodist, hairdresser, local clergy, mobile library and a local WRVS 'sweet trolley', together with outside trips to the optician, dentist or merely for shopping. Observations in the main lounge revealed that when the staff have finished 'their work', they invariably sat together with the residents in one place and the staff in another. Clearly, the staff require a rest and a 'break' from constant interaction with residents. Having to constantly carry out what Smith (1992) describes as *'emotional labour'*, dealing with the psychological needs of residents within a confined setting can be exhausting. From my previous research studies in hospitals and hospices, this seems to be a feature of many institutional settings particularly where older people are the client group. Newlands was no exception. Care staff were however discouraged from spending time in the office away from the main resident area, although this did not apply to managers. Observing residents is always important should they experience sudden cardiovascular problems (fits, strokes and heart attacks). This is important when residents may be at increased risk from falls, particularly residents with dementia.

Staffing issues

Residential homes differ greatly in their internal structure as well as their policies and practices. Many of the staff are not well paid and there are limited training opportunities and little scope for career development. There is also great variation in the standards of care and the management of residents (Peace et al 1997). The research on staffing levels in residential care homes suggests that staff in a number of homes lack specific training in communication skills and bereavement care (Sidell et al 1997). In many ways dealing with dying residents and supporting the relatives in their grief is a major challenge and source of stress for the staff in many residential homes. The all-female staff consisted of one manager, two deputy managers, nine care assistants, two cooks and one domestic. During my visit one cook had left and this meant that the care staff took turns to double up as cook. The cook's job was to provide meals for all the residents including day residents and at weekends to provide up to 15 'meals on wheels' for local older people. The care assistants did receive a wide range of training in moving and handling, food hygiene, first aid and various NVQ refresher training courses. Residents' views were sought on a range of matters relating to the quality of service provided. Staffing issues were raised by residents along with food, night time noise levels, laundry and a number of domestic issues. On the whole the residents views (published on the main notice board) were largely favourable.

Different models of care

Historically, institutional care for older people has been described as emanating from two distinct models of care, the warehousing model and the horticultural model (Miller & Gwynne 1972). The former is associated with hospital care and the aim of prolonging physical life by representing attempts to translate the model into residential contexts. The defining features of the patient are their physical, emotional and social needs for care. In the hospital setting, curative approaches which fail are often reflected in the nurses' sense of failure when a patient dies, particularly in critical care contexts (Field 1984, Seymour 2001). Newlands was unable to provide the type of medical care closely associated with warehousing due to the lack of nursing and medical provision. However the staff, often unconsciously, fostered a sense of dependence and depersonalisation in residents when they could have adopted a more empowering approach to facilitate change and a sense of independence in the residents. Anecdotal evidence suggests that nurses are not unaware of the way in which nursing care can depersonalise patients and refer to this process as 'sheep dipping'. Rather than initiate a shopping trip into the local town, care staff would bring in individual items for residents. Although a shopping trip did takes place, they were very few and far between. Staff at Newlands often saw the resident as spending the rest of their lives there and their role was protective and paternal.

In contrast, the horticultural model is aimed at enabling residents to develop independence and foster a sense of hope and well-being for their independent future. Admission to a residential centre operating the horticultural model would see physical care as a constraint. The resident is perceived as an individual with ability, who because of their circumstances is unable to function effectively due to unfulfilled capacities. The nurse's role is to develop these capacities and actively engage in rehabilitation. This is an issue taken up by Kellehear (1999) in relation to the palliative care needs of patients with life threatening medical illness. Both models of care are evident in hospitals and other institutional settings. The care at Newlands reflected both types of approach. Wherever possible staff would urge residents to wash and dress themselves and make their own way to and from the toilet and dining areas. However, when the routine was disrupted due to shortages of staff the staff would revert to a more warehouse way of ensuring that the key tasks of washing, dressing eating and drinking were carried out within a particular time frame.

Talking about death and dying

Death was not a regular occurrence at Newlands with a maximum of four deaths a year. This compares well with figures from Counsel and Care (1995). The general philosophy of the staff regarding resident longevity was that many residents would not live as long as they did if they were not in residential care:

> We look after them well, feed them well, care for their physical and psychological needs and generally make sure they come to no harm. One of the most awful things is when a resident outlives their children.

One of the interesting features of the assessment and admission of residents was the question asked on the assessment form regarding preferences about management of their body after death. On admission to Newlands, the assessment form requires that the prospective residents (or their families) determine, in the event of their death, whether they would prefer to be cremated or buried.

When a death takes place, residents and staff who wish to attend the funeral are encouraged to do so. In particular, residents were keen to pay their respects by donating to the flowers sent to the family on their behalf.

The death of a resident

When residents died at Newlands, staff were not allowed to confirm death, which was the prerogative of the resident's GP. Once the GP had visited and confirmed death, the family were then informed and asked what arrangements they had made, or would like making about the funeral and if they had a preferred funeral director. Often this information was included in the resident's care plan and the staff were able to contact the appropriate funeral director and ask them to remove the body. The funeral director would arrive at Newlands and using their discretion remove the deceased resident in a body bag, often entering and leaving via the rear entrance.

Residents were informed when someone died and often this was expected and residents asked how they were progressing. With the exception of the question about cremation or burial during the residents admission, discussion of death and dying was muted and apart from when a resident was actually dying, little was said. I did ask a number of residents about their attitude towards death and although most were happy to share their thoughts, there was more than a hint of fatalism in their responses:

> Well, folk get ill and they are poorly, some manage to get through it and others well they don't and I suppose they die and that's it.

This seemed to reflect the general attitude towards death at Newlands. If a resident shows signs of illness they often remained in their room, although not always in bed. The care manager calls the GP if necessary. Isolation is used to prevent the spread of any infection (a wise precaution in such settings). Concern with physical care is demonstrated through the use of soap and water pressure area care despite nursing research suggesting that this is to be avoided (see Waterlow 1988). Hydration and nutrition are also important features of the care, ensuring that poorly residents are looked after, although no intravenous lines or specific nursing equipment are used. Should a resident require hospitalisation this is arranged in a similar way to them being at home. The patient is cared for and given tender loving care (TLC), until such time as they recover or die. Residents who ask about their deceased friend are told and allowed to pay their respects if they wish, although no specific ritual takes place for this to happen.

The residents of Newlands attended the funerals and memorial services of friends and family members. Acknowledging death and ensuring that last respects are observed are important parts of the social activity especially for older people in institutional settings (Costello 1996).

Social death

The term social death is derived from a pilot study of institutional life for physically handicapped individuals sponsored by the then Ministry of Health between 1966 and 1969 (Miller & Gwynne 1972). The study made an important contribution to our understanding of institutional processes. Since that time, a number of authors from different disciplines have described the latter period of life for some very old people as a transition through social death to clinical death. Social death is seen to occur for certain types of people: the terminally ill, the very old, and those who have lost their essential personhood (i.e. due to Persistent Vegetative State or severe dementia or learning disabilities) (Sweeting & Gilhooley 1991). In this sense the attributes that help to make up the person and provide them with a worthwhile life often referred to as 'personhood' are limited and in some cases non-existent. When this takes place, the term social death may be used to denote a situation where there is no easily discernible social contact between the person and the outside world. We can argue about what makes up personhood and a worthwhile life, although it is clear that without meaningful social contact, it is reasonable to speculate that there is a loss in the person's social repertoire. The types of people regarded as experiencing social death are often the very old who live in institutional settings. Some authors have argued that old age and natural death are linked and that as many old people are expected to die, their passage towards death may involve a degree of social death, since they have earned the right to die (Kastenbaum 1995). This perception is reinforced when the older person lives in an institutional setting, has few if any visitors and suffers from advanced dementia. Their daily contact with others is limited to the staff and other residents (who may be in a similar situation to themselves). This did not apply to most residents of Newlands, although for some, social death appeared to be an accurate description of their daily lives. It is interesting to examine what helps to make up social death in an institutional setting. First, the atmosphere at Newlands was quiet and often unstimulating apart from social occasions. The majority of residents invariably sat in the same chairs each day with a few exceptions such as those mobile enough to transfer themselves from the main lounge, into the non-smoking lounge or the vestibule area that contained a conservatory. A very small number of residents preferred to spend time alone in their bedrooms, coming out to attend meals and occasionally sit in the main lounge. Alice made the point:

> ... we're all alive aren't we, but nobody speaks. What we
> need is more entertainment, now that would be a good idea.
> Nothing much happens here. We occasionally lose a cus-
> tomer or two [In this instance she was referring not to death
> but to loss of social contact due to Alzheimer's disease.]

When using the term social death, I am attempting to convey an
image of life at Newlands for some residents, but not all. Two
things need to be considered about the notion of social death.
First that it is important to consider that social death may occur
gradually through a range of actions including attempts to pro-
tect residents from being upset by outside stimulation such as the
death of a friend. Secondly, social death is not inevitable. Focused
social interaction, an orientation towards residents and a genuine
culture of care can prevent the features of social death becoming
an embedded part of institutional life. Goffman (1968) used the
term mortification to denote the ways in which institutions provided barriers to social interaction. This included things such as
limiting visitors, being geographically placed at the margins of
communities and by having a *'limited round of activity'* in other
words sleep, rest and play all take place in a confined area. There
is a need therefore for such settings to become as open as possible, inviting outsiders to enter and engage in any way possible
with the residents. There is also a need to facilitate the residents
to interact with each other and develop a social culture that is
maintained and developed through mutual agreements and tacit
conventions.

Martha

Martha, was a 91 year old widow, who had been a resident for
16 months following admission due to immobility and as a result
of a series of falls at home, where she lived alone. The following
is the transcript of a short 20 minute conversation with her in the
non-smoking lounge at Newlands. Despite her age Martha was
mentally alert and very quick witted, she was not slow to criticise
and was unhappy about losing her independence on having to be
admitted.

JC: What is it that you like about Newlands?

Martha: Nothing, nothing at all.

JC: Nothing at all, surely you like something?

Martha: No, nothing

JC: How do you find the food?

Martha: Yes well it's alright I suppose, but it's not like living at home and making your own how you want it is it?

JC: Yes true but is it not nice to have someone cook for you?

Martha: In a way yes but I still prefer to be in my own bungalow with someone looking after me in my own place.

JC: How long were you living in your bungalow?

Martha: Twenty years on me own, ee it was lonely at times though and I suppose not very nice some of the time but it was my own.

JC: Do you consider it an advantage now to have people around you?

Martha: No! 'cos there's not one in 'ere you can have a decent conversation with, either they're asleep, deaf or talk rubbish most 'ot time if you get me meaning.

JC: Well, I've managed to have some good chats with people around here what about … Alice here (gestures to the lady in the next chair).

Martha: Give over thee half of 'em here well I don't know they're as daft as a brush. During the day some of 'em are alright, Alice and I have a natter don't we but at night oh God, night time it's like a mad 'ouse in 'ere at time. There's her over there never stops screaming the place down. I can natter with Alice but at times I canna make out what she's saying. [Alice has had a stroke.]

At this stage it was tea time and Martha moved over to the table for her evening meal.

Alice

Alice was a 91 year old widow who had been admitted to Newlands 11 months previously because 'I was not able to look after myself.' Alice had tried other homes and spent 3 weeks in an assessment centre but had not liked 'the atmosphere' of the other places. During the 3 week period of assessment it became clear that her main problem was a lack of mobility due to arthritis. Alice was also suffering from Alzheimer's disease and became forgetful, particularly about time, with characteristic recent memory loss. This meant that she was able to function quite well and recall events of the past much better than recent ones. Alice could not recall when she was admitted to Newlands but remembered that her husband died in 1968, they had no children and Alice described her life as being a very happy one. After her husband's death, she lived alone in local council accommodation. Alice had worked in the local mills as a spinner and weaver since she left school at the age of 14 'I liked working in the mill it was hard at times but we managed to enjoy us selves'. Alice was very clear about what she thought about Newlands:

> It's very nice here I like it a lot, the place is very clean and tidy and I enjoy the food and the people (staff and other residents) are very nice and well mannered, yes I do I like it here very much, no I like it, it's nice and quiet.

In terms of contact with outsiders, Alice was visited regularly by her cousin and occasionally by a friend who lived locally.

Natural death or ageism?

One of the features of care at Newlands was the attitude of the staff and residents towards death, dying and bereavement. Residents expressed concern for those who died and sympathy for relatives, but death was not a major source of stress. One care manager pointed out that:

> Residents do die although not very often, we haven't had a death now for nearly a year and when Ellen died it was expected although if you ask the residents they are not likely to remember her passing.

I asked two residents about anyone they knew who had died. Both recalled that there had been a death in the last year but could not remember who. I had a sense that death was not a major event and that although many residents were aware of their vulnerability in terms of being 'close to death', it was not discussed at any length. As one resident put it: 'I know that I am going to die, aren't we all? But there's no sense in worrying about it, you have to live each day as it comes'. In many ways resident and staff attitudes towards death support the view of others who argue that societal ageism tends to devalue older people in general compared with younger people (Scrutton 1995, Moss & Moss 1996). In many ways the idea that it is natural for old people to die has become a theme within our society. Of course it is natural for us to die when we get old since in one way, death and old age go together, we all have to die and as a nurse, I and others have experienced the relief when an older patient has died, because it meant a form of release, 'a blessing'. Kastenbaum (1995) points out that one of the problems with the attitude that it is natural to die when you are old, is that it can de-value the impact of death and minimalise its importance to older people. Once older people begin to think of death as a valueless event, then others such as carers will become persuaded to think of death as having limited importance.

Denial of death

It may be argued that coping with life is about coping with the fact of death. For many residents death was not unfamiliar and as death approached they developed ways of living with the fact of death. Peace & Katz (2003) ask whether the denial of death by people in care homes is the ultimate ageism?

One response to this could be that if older people are intimately involved in and remain close to death, then denying it may be seen as a way of 'creating a space' to not think about it. The logical progression of this argument is that the process of dying may be seen as a 'normal' step towards what is considered to be the inevitable. However, dying can be a long drawn out process involving much suffering and distress for the person and those who share this period of crisis. My observations of staff and resident attitudes at Newlands did not lead me to believe that the staff were either 'ageist' or unconcerned about death and dying. On reflection, the attitudes of the staff and residents towards death reflected the context in which it took place. Death was often 'hidden from view'; it was not explicit and did not take centre stage. Death happened, it was spoken about, but in whispers rather than calling a general meeting! This did not demonstrate any tangible form of 'death denial'. Moreover, death was considered a sad but natural occurrence and the staff got on with doing what they needed to do in terms of grooming the patient, preparing the body for collection by the funeral director and offering their sympathies to the grieving relatives. In short, death was another event in the lives of residents that needed to be managed and 'got over', so that residents and staff could get on with their everyday lives.

Caring for residents with dementia

The history of care for residents in residential settings varies with adverse comment citing neglect, maltreatment, inadequate support and the overuse of drugs to sedate older people. It is however important not to draw too much from the many negative views made about the care of residents with dementia. The Alzheimer's Society (1997) conducted a survey of experiences of care in residential settings aimed at residents' partners/relatives. The evidence indicates that 85% of carers were reasonably happy about the level of care and described it as 'satisfactory' with 70% rating food, staff attitudes and physical environment highly. However, in 10% of cases, the care was said to be poor or average for personal aspects of care with 49% reporting a lack of GP support and 10% citing evidence of maltreatment.

Keady (1997) asks how carers can subjectively describe the care process so highly, when they are aware that the 'lived realities of care' for residents are so poor with instances of neglect, lack of staff support and a poor level of training for care staff. Keady postulates that perhaps the relatives are in a form of denial which masks the guilt they feel because they are unable to care for their loved one themselves. This is a reasonable assumption, although in practice it is perhaps more useful to consider the other possibilities.

Summary

A number of studies have considered quality of life for older people in residential settings, although few have focused specifically on the experiences of death and dying (Ford & Heath 1996, Froggatt et al 2001). This chapter, through a consideration of the care in one setting has examined the wider dimensions of death namely social death and its effects on older residents. The social structures within Newlands were constructed from within the institution. It would be inaccurate to suggest that the staff were the sole contributors to the culture of care. Moreover, the residents formed an important part of everyday life and contributed towards supporting other residents. Despite this, there was also much evidence of the 'warehousing model' of care being adopted whereby the primary task becomes the prolongation of life and the transference of hospital-type routines into the residential context. The rules and conventions were largely constructed through staff discourses. There were similarities with the hierarchical order of the hospital although, a more egalitarian approach was evident in the way residents organised their daily lives. In this sense the type of 'resident dependency' typical of the warehousing model was not as evident as it would be in hospital settings. There were fewer power struggles taking place between different occupational groups. There was also a blurring of roles as many people swapped roles and were able to 'act up and down' according to need (care assistants may become cooks or assistant matrons). In this sense, the care providers were able to establish their own norms and act as 'agents' in making a difference to the way in which care was provided. As a population, the residents suffered from a range of chronic illnesses both physical and psychological. The culture of care and the attitudes of the staff quite often reflected those of wider society (Hockey 1990). Social ageism along with other issues such as staff shortages, lack of resources, attitudes towards social death, skill mix and staff competence and the routinisation of care, influence the quality of life and the provision of what may be called a good death in residential care. Unlike other settings in which death may be seen as a threat or a stigmatised occurrence, my observations and discussions at Newlands led me to consider that death was perceived by staff and residents as an everyday event which will affect all residents at some time or another. This contrasts with the attitudes of nurses in some hospital contexts such as ICU where death was associated with a sense of failure (Field 1989).

In relation to the future of death and dying in nursing and residential care homes, two things are clear. First, that it is likely we

will see an increased number of older dying people in these settings. Secondly as Field & Froggatt (2003) point out it is likely
that we will see the development of palliative care outside of
hospitals and hospices due to a series of political, social and
professional influences on the care of older people in community
settings. The observations from Newlands, whilst not generalisable,
have perhaps contributed toward the wider debate concerning the
need to focus attention on the care of older people in residential
care. In particular, the issues and challenges which face residents
and staff at the end of life.

Further reading

Froggatt K., Hoult L. & Poole K. (2001) *Community work with nursing
and residential care homes: a survey study of clinical nurse specialists in
palliative care.* Macmillan Cancer Relief/The Institute of Cancer Research,
London.

This research report provides an overview of the role of specialist nurses
which involves providing advice and support for practitioners in residential and nursing home settings. The report gives a very useful account of
the provision of care in this important area for the future, including an
examination of the education and training needs of care staff and their
relationship with specialist practitioners.

Katz J.S. & Peace S. (2003) *End of life in care homes: a palliative care
approach.* Oxford University Press, Oxford.

This well-written book provides a comprehensive account of the care
provided in nursing and residential care homes. There are 12 chapters
written by nine very experienced contributors who focus attention on a
wide range of issues; from who dies in care homes, to an examination of
the key palliative care issues. The authors explain what palliative care is
and some of the challenges and successes for developing a palliative care
approach in nursing homes. The book also considers the role of external
agencies and specialist nurses and the need for staff training and education. It is more a text book and provides a rich overview of the social,
political and cultural dimensions of care.

Miller E.J. & Gwynne G.V. (1972) *A life apart: a pilot study of residential institutions for the physically handicapped and the very young sick.*
Tavistock Books, London.

This is a classic text recommended by the Open University as a required
reading material for those involved in the care of people with learning

disabilities. Although this is not a book about death and dying, the authors conduct a rigorous analysis of care organisation and the ways in which staff and patients cope with their everyday lives. The book examines social attitudes and the link between those living within institutions and those on the outside.

Peace S., Kellaher L. & Willcocks D. (1997) *Re-evaluating residential care.* Open University Press, Buckingham.

This book takes a critical look at the provision of care in residential settings and attempts to contrast the internal social structures of residential care with the social attitudes of wider society towards older people. A number of issues are raised including ageism and attitudes of older people towards death and dying and the use of denial of death as a coping strategy.

Part IV
Caring in a community context

The final part of the book consists of two chapters. Chapter 8 focuses on the care of terminally ill patients in their own home and the role of the community nursing team in providing care at the end of life. The chapter offers a personal view of my Father's death and the care he received in the last year of his life spent in our family home. Chapter 9 reflects back on the conclusions from each chapter and examines the way in which death and dying over the last two decades has become medicalised and traces the shift away from family care to institutional care. This final chapter considers the impact death has on the family in terms of grief and bereavement and considers the concept of 'dying well' and the things that nurses and others can do to ensure the patient has a 'good death'.

8 Death and dying in the community

Introduction

In the first half of the last century most deaths in the UK occurred at home, although by the 1960s this was reduced to one-third, with figures suggesting that about a quarter of all cancer patients and one-fifth of all deaths are at home (Higginson et al 1998). It is well known that although most deaths in Britain occur in hospital, the majority of terminal care takes place in the home and much of the palliative care is undertaken by lay carers (often women), who are relatives of the dying person (Seale & Cartwright 1994). The vast majority of doctors and nurses I speak to about death and dying point out that given the choice, the vast majority prefer to die at home. This in itself, reflects much of the negativity surrounding the experience of death and dying in institutional care. The patient's GP, community nurses as well as the human and material resources available to the family, play a significant part in the provision of care provided at home.

The purpose of this chapter is to describe the care provided to people who receive terminal care and die at home. What follows is a description and evaluation of how dying at home presents opportunities for the dying person to be cared for in an all too familiar environment, as well as examining the many potential problems that can take place when it is decided to care for a loved one in the home. Accounts of the experiences of professional and lay carers' perspectives are examined. To illustrate many of the issues raised by community nurses, a personalised account is included of the terminal care received by my Father during his last year within our family home until his eventual expected death in 1988.

It is perhaps no surprise to find that when asked about where they would like to die the vast majority of people in the UK and elsewhere, state that they want to die at home (Seale & Cartwright 1994, Wilson 2000). The chapter will attempt to address why there is an increasing trend towards death taking place in hospital, if so many people prefer home deaths (Higginson et al 2002), and 22% of hospital beds are taken up by people in the last year of their life.

Why die at home?

Historically, with the exception of war, people have always died at home. The idea that anyone would wish to die outside the security of their own home would have been unheard of. When you consider the reputation that hospitals have over the years why would anyone really want to go into a hospital to die? In contemporary times however, for all kinds of reasons, the decision to be cared for and die at home is not an easy one and there are many reasons why people choose to leave it to the professionals. For some patients, dying at home satisfies a desire to be amongst loves ones and for the experience to be a positive one, it needs to be matched by the carer's ability to provide the right type of care, sustained in many cases, for long periods of time. As Appleton (1995) points out:

> The decision to share the very end of life in a family setting is one of the highest acts of love that any of us can ever hope to experience.

Traditionally, terminal care equated with family care. Clark (1993) provides an excellent description of the way in which members of the family and the local community at the turn of the 20th century managed death in a small seaside town in the North of England. Since then, the tradition of family care has become more limited since death and dying became medicalised and professionalised in contemporary society. Instead of the clergy attending the dying person, now it is often medical staff or more accurately, nurses. The modern funeral director now plays a large role in managing the affairs at the end of life. This includes relieving the family and friends of much of the 'emotional labour' involved at the end of life, but at the same time preventing the family from becoming involved in the necessary preparatory work which can help them to cope with the death (Walter 1990). More recently, it has become a central feature of government policy to try and enable people to die in the community with a wide range of settings providing palliative, terminal and respite care. These include hospices, day centres, nursing homes and residential homes for older people. A consequence of this push towards care in the community has been the pressure placed on domiciliary services, in particular community nursing to provide terminal care (Seale & Cartwright 1994).

Terminal care has often been reserved for the specific care of the dying patient who reached an advanced state where dying is likely in the very near future and is in the last stages of life. In contemporary terms the care given to those who are known to be on a dying 'trajectory' is also known as supportive care with palliative care used more often when referring to specialist services such as clinical nurse specialists or medical practitioners. Consistent with all aspects of palliation, the care provided extends to the patient and the family. The latter in some cases becomes the focus of the practitioner's attention, when for example the patient's condition is stabilised and the emotional needs of the family become a priority. Caring for a terminally ill person at home can be a daunting task and a number of factors are involved in enabling the person to die what many would consider a good death at home (see Figure 8.1).

- Support from the primary care team.
- Practical issues.
- Involvement of specialists, i.e. Macmillan/Marie Curie nurses.
- The health and well being of the primary caregivers.

Figure 8.1   Factors involved in caring for dying people at home

Support from the primary care team

Since the publication of the Standing Medical Advisory Committee in 1980 which stated that the best, as well as the worst terminal care can take place at home, attention has been placed on how to best support families and patients who are dying at home. Various guidelines suggesting ways in which terminal care in the UK can be improved in the home setting advocate for strong links to be made between the family and professional care givers, with particular emphasis being placed on communication (King Edward's Hospital Fund for London & National Association of Health Authorities and Trusts 1991, Scottish Home Office & Health Department 1991).

One of the key players in determining the quality of terminal care at home is the GP. The main difference between the care hospital staff provided and the type of care and treatment provided by the GP was in the nature of the relationship between GP and patient. This is a view supported by Field (1998) who points out that GPs caring for dying patients saw themselves as a team and invariably had a relationship with the patient prior to the development of their terminal illness. They were also likely to know the family and have insight into their wishes and preferences for treatment. This was certainly the case when my Father was dying at home and it became clear that we did not want his life to be prolonged unnecessarily by continuing treatment, when it was not felt (by the family) to be appropriate. Having a good relationship with the GP prior to my Father living with us meant that we were able to discuss this sensitive matter safe in the knowledge that the GP had a reasonable understanding of our views and was able to sympathise with our dilemma. I am not sure that the matter could have been dealt with anywhere near as well with someone who had no prior knowledge of the family or a clear idea of our intentions towards my Father.

The care provided by the GP and the primary care team plays a key role in enabling the family to cope at home during a very stressful time. Health centre receptionists and practice nurses also play a role in supporting (by not intruding/intruding on) the family, for example facilitating them to obtain medication at short notice and booking prompt appointments where necessary. These small things can and do make a difference when the family are finding the situation at home difficult to deal with.

Nursing care of the dying patient at home

The caseload of most community nurses will include patients who are approaching death. In conducting the research to this book,

I spoke with many community nurses about their role in caring for dying patients. This section includes a number of comments and contributions from nurses working in a busy inner city practice where care at the end of life was not unusual and never routine. Dying patients are often clearly known to district nurses who provide high quality 24-hour care within the resources available to them. Families or partners who express a wish to care for a dying relative in their own home will receive care from qualified nurses experienced in the care of dying patients. The provision of care at the end of life when a patient is dying at home includes the contribution of Marie Curie nurses. These professional nurses and health support workers, very experienced in terminal care, give support at night and in some cases will stay in the patient's home overnight, providing a night sitting service. Macmillan nurses may also become involved, especially when the patient has a cancer diagnosis. District nurses invariably try to introduce the patient to all members of the team by carrying out visits in teams of two:

> It is difficult sometimes for nurses to know the family, so we visit terminal patients in twos at different times, often we make two visits a day using different nurses.

The focus of much of the district nurse's work is the prevention and control of symptoms such as pain, nausea and vomiting, breathlessness and fatigue. Needless to say patients experience much more than physical symptoms. Invariably, nurses find it difficult to be specific about their role in providing community based care to dying patients:

> It is very hard to say specifically what our role is with terminal care patients, often it is a question of controlling pain, but this nearly always involves supporting the carer and providing a listening ear.

Patients referred for district nursing care by GPs, receive attention on a needs basis. That is, nurses carry out an initial assessment based on what the patient requires and then negotiate with the family the best way to meet these needs. One district nurse pointed out that:

> I often find it useful to work out what families want first
> and then try as best as I can to arrive at the house when
> they need me.

Patients requiring continuous pain relief are often provided with
a syringe driver, which delivers pain relief and anti emetic medication simultaneously through the driver. District nurses will often
'top up' the syringe driver over a 24-hour basis, with night calls
being made to the patient.

> The night staff will be informed if there are patients receiv-
> ing terminal care at home even if it is a case of being aware
> that there is a terminal patient but they don't need a call at
> night because quite often they die at night.

Negotiating the input from the district nursing team is problematic
since the needs of the patient vary and it is not always possible to
ensure continuity of care within the district nursing team because
of demand, shift variations and availability of individual nurses.

> We like to get to know those families where there is a dying
> patient but it is not always possible and sometimes we have
> to do a visit to cover a colleague or when we are not entirely
> familiar with the patient.

Community nurses provide much more than pain relief and symptom control since many patients will have a range of co-morbidities
such as in-dwelling catheters, leg ulcers and wound dressings. In
some cases, the nurse may be required to carry out specific nursing duties such as the giving of an insulin injection, or changing
a dressing. In other cases, the nurse will carry out washing and
dressing as well as management of continence and continence
aids. Patients with MS and MND often require substantial assistance from more than one nurse:

> In some cases two nurses are required to work the hoist
> and to make sure the patient does not experience more
> pain and discomfort, this is possible by managing and

coordinating our respective workloads although at night, it is much harder to do.

Most nurses caring for dying patients at home are well aware of the enormous burden placed on primary carers. Finding time to offer a listening ear and the necessary psychological support places a strain on district nursing services:

> Let's face it, a visit to a terminally ill patient is more than just a dressing change and oftentimes, before you get to the patient you need to spend time with the carer explaining what's going on advising them on practical things and just listening to their worries.

Enabling patients to die with dignity at home is a major challenge to district nursing teams. In many cases families become very dependent on nursing support, especially where there is equipment involved. This can be the cause of a number of stressors:

> We do get a lot of calls about problems with patients and carers being worried about syringe drivers and calls from relatives about the patients' level of pain.

Such 'crisis calls' need to be responded to quickly and often a visit will be required, although if the family and the nurse have a good relationship, a phone call from the patient's nurse can often reassure the patient and a visit can be planned that enables the nurse to continue with his/her other visits:

> Personally I like caring for dying people at home, but if I am honest, I don't always have the time to do it properly. I know we all say that, but sometimes you feel torn between spending more time with the dying patients at the expense of others, whose needs are often as great, but they are not dying.

One of the key issues in caring for dying patients at home is the provision of pain relief using syringe drivers. Families have the responsibility for collecting controlled drugs (or may have an arrangement with pharmacies for delivery), and the nurse will check the dose, record what is given on a patient's drug card and prime the syringe driver for a 24-hour period. Nurses do not carry controlled drugs, which is strictly enforced especially since the Dr Shipman case. The interventions made by district nurses are documented on two sets of notes. One set is kept in the home so that different nurses who make unscheduled visits are able to see what others have carried out. Another set of notes is kept in the district nursing office.

Difficulties in providing terminal care at home

Not all death in the community is expected and sometimes patients die suddenly without district nurse input. There are also problems associated with the timing of 'out of hours' deaths, when patients die on bank holidays and weekends. In such cases, emergency doctors may become involved through the 'Go to Doc' system outside of normal surgery times. This involves a locum GP visiting or providing advice to a distressed family faced with the sudden death of a loved one. One of the problems of using 'Go to Doc' services is that if a patient has not been seen by their GP within the last two weeks, the patient's death is referred to the Coroner since the GP is not allowed to sign the death certificate. A post mortem takes place and invariably the police become involved. This is largely as a result of the Dr Shipman case and is an attempt to ensure that the patient died from natural causes. To minimise trauma to the family, district nurses when aware of the patient's imminent death, facilitate a home visit by the GP who is then able to sign the death certificate.

Another major challenge, is the timing of a patient's death and their specific need for care and treatment. Many teams work until 17.00 hours with the next shift starting at 18.00 hours. Whilst nurses would not allow the needs of a patient to go unmet, invariably, the timing of a call for pain relief or to 'top up' a syringe driver may occur when nursing availability is limited. Another related problem is when a patient dies at a weekend or a bank holiday. The latter are particularly problematic because of the reduced number of staff on duty and many difficulties arise when patients require specific advice and help with pain control:

Weekends are a problem sometimes for providing the best type of care for dying patients, mainly because GP and district nurse input is reduced. From the families' point of view, pain relief on a Sunday afternoon can become frustrating and on Monday morning there are often problems to resolve because of weekend hassles.

It is difficult to convey a truly accurate picture of the type of care patients receive from community nurses in all areas. Each region throughout the country will have a set of protocols which will vary according to local issues, such as geographical constraints faced by nurses in rural areas and problems associated with carrying out care in inner city areas, where home visits may be hampered by the need for security resulting from areas of high crime. In themselves these contextual issues impinge on the ability of the health professionals to ensure that dying patients receive high, consistent levels of care.

Community nurses and the family

One of the key factors in terms of the quality of a death at home is the interrelationship between the community nurses and the family. The evidence suggests that although the care of dying people at home has improved in the last 20 years there is still room for improvement (Jones et al 1993). In Jones et al's study, the 207 carers would have liked more advice about help available outside of the hospital, in particular help with domestic work. There were also complaints that carers' problems were not given sufficient attention. From a personal perspective, I found the nurses very helpful in caring for my Father but less focused on the needs of my family. This may be due to the fact that my wife and I were both in the health care profession, although the evidence suggests that carers' problems are less of an issue since they are not the ones who need the help, until it comes to bereavement support after death.

Gaining insight into the needs of dying people and their relatives is a complex issue. Copp (1999:132) describes the way in which dying people juggle with their thoughts in relation to public and private dimensions. The latter she describes as being more complex and involves several layers depending on the individual. The 'public front' was kept at a more superficial level and only when there was a fracture of the public and private dimensions, for example when the person made a public expression but privately there were underlying tensions. An example of this is the fear of dying. Many people not facing death make bold statements about death alluding to a lack of fear. However, when the time of death occurs many feel a type of anxiety related to the fact that they have not seriously considered their own feelings. I recall informing colleagues at work that I was not worried about my Dad's death since I had reached the point (I felt) that death was inevitable. When he died however, I was surprised at how worried I was (fearing my own expression of feelings) and how sad it made me feel.

Dying at home: practical issues

Supporting people dying at home raises a number of emotional, physical and psychological problems as well as placing a financial strain on families in terms of meeting the multiple needs of the dying person. There are a range of resources available to help meet the financial burden, including benefits to offset, but by no means meet all the costs of care in the home. According to Lee (1995) 85% of patients with cancer receive no financial help at all and those with non-malignant disease do not fare much better. Added to this the experience of illness and hospitalisation can be an expensive one, not only in terms of loss of earnings but also the cost of travelling to and from hospital (for which financial support can be gained) and also the 'human cost' of having a loved one in a place perceived to be a strange environment.

Attendance allowance is paid to people whose care needs begin after the 65th birthday and who cannot get Disability Living Allowance (DLA). In normal circumstances the patient needs to have care needs for 6 months although this does not apply to terminally ill people who have what is called special circumstances. There are two rates of attendance allowance: the lower rate and the higher rate. The former is paid if the person needs attention with personal care frequently throughout the day. This care has to be in connection with bodily functions such as washing, dressing, bathing and toilet needs and help taking medication. The higher rate is paid to patients who are terminally ill with a life expectancy of 6 months or less. It is also paid to people who are not terminally ill but require attention during the night and day to manage the activities of daily living previously described. To apply for attendance allowance you are required to complete the form in leaflet DS702 available from social security offices, social workers, or if in residential care, the staff are often able to obtain this on the patient's behalf.

Disability Living Allowance is a non-means tested benefit paid to people, including children, under 65 years of age who are unable or have difficulty carrying out activities of daily living and is paid on top of other existing benefits. Normally the person must have had care needs for at least 3 months, unless they are terminally ill and must be needing the help for a further 6 months. It is not possible to claim DLA on or after your 65th birthday. The benefit is paid at three rates, with a mobility component used for helping the person get around which is paid at two rates. The lowest rate is paid to those who only need a small amount of help each day, such as getting dressed or paid to people who cannot make a meal if they are given all the ingredients (must be over the age of 16). The mobility component is paid to people who can walk but need someone to guide them in places, which are unfamiliar (low rate). The higher rate applies to people who have severe difficulty with walking because of pain or severe discomfort. Details about all benefits can be obtained from social work departments, local post offices as well as through publications such as 'A guide to benefits' Dept of Social Security (2000).

Help in the home

The decision to care for someone at home who is expected to die requires a clear assessment of what is involved other than the emotional issues. First, are the resources at the disposal of the family and their ability to utilise them. For some people, despite preferences, the choice of where to die is an issue determined by the family and is largely based on practical considerations and whether they feel they can manage the patient's problems (Jones 1992). Living in a small house with limited space is a key factor, although with the help of occupational therapists, physiotherapists, nurses and doctors and in some cases, surveyors, the practical problems can be alleviated. Adaptations to the home, e.g. a stair rail, raised toilet seat or a house extension, not only ensures greater comfort but also increases quality of care and much less work for the care providers, both the family and the community nurses.

One of the key issues facing carers at home is their ability to provide their loved one with a high standard of care. A major consideration is the question – can I look after them properly? Smith (1994) reports that many nurses anxious to support older people on being discharged home expressed doubts about the ability of the patient and relative to cope due to the carer's physical impairments. A number of other factors suggest that the prospect of caring for dying people presents many challenges for families. Evidence suggests that there is a lack of resources and skills in the community to support dying patients and their families (Cartwright 1991), although, more recent evidence suggests that this situation is changing. Government guidelines (Department of Health 2000a) indicate that Primary Care Trusts should provide greater levels of support for families who wish to care for family members in the home setting. The role of the primary care team and in particular community nurses is central to effective terminal care in the home.

Community occupational therapist involvement

An important member of the multi-disciplinary team in the community who can offer support and practical help is the occupational therapist (OT). The OT forms part of the Social Services team and focuses on patients with a wide range of difficulties, which render them unable to carry out their normal activities of living. The role of the OT is to assess patients and attempt to ensure maximum independence or to maintain and improve their quality of life. For dying patients this often translates as providing them with practical aids to assist them in carrying out activities of daily living and to supplement the work of nurses. This can include providing equipment and aids to assist with washing and dressing or the provision of extra rails on steps and stairs. OTs often provide other professionals, as well as patients and families with advice on ways to reduce the problems of carrying out everyday activity when illness prevents independence. In particular OTs can provide equipment such as chair risers, grab rails, raised toilet seats and appropriate beds, although often nurses are able to obtain

NHS type beds. OTs are also able to provide ramps to enable easy access and even stair lifts. In some cases, where the patient's quality of life could be improved with major changes, OTs can initiate the building of an extension, the installation of a vertical lift/stair lift and the provision of an additional toilet in the house. To be eligible for such help, an application needs to be made to Social Services and a request for a visit. To be eligible for assistance with home adaptations, a patient must be substantially and permanently incapacitated. Patients in advanced stages of MS and MND are often those who can gain maximum support through the provision of home adaptations. Anyone, including the patient, district nurses, social workers and GPs can make the referral for an OT assessment. An OT visit is usually prioritised and patients with life threatening illnesses will receive a high priority. The OT will carry out an assessment of needs and discuss possible solutions with the patient and family. OTs liaise closely with nurses and can often facilitate increased independence and directly support the care providers. OT support can involve a cost although advice is free. Each Social Services OT department can levy charges for their practical help. As a general rule, adaptations under £1000 (the figure in my area) are free of charge. For those over £1000, it is necessary to apply for disabled grant facilities, which is subject to financial assessment. OTs are happy to provide full and comprehensive advice on how to obtain financial support.

Involvement of specialist nurses

The vast majority of people who have benefited from their services often hold Macmillan nurses and other specialist palliative and cancer specialists such as Marie Curie nurses in high regard. Others however find the idea of such people tinged with the thought of death and make statements such as 'Oh No I don't want them round', reflecting that for some, Macmillan nurses equate with death. The involvement of Macmillan nurses in the care of the terminally ill patient either in hospital or the community is based on a referral system. Macmillan nurses do not impose their services on people, instead they are asked by other professionals for their advice and are often available for patients and families at the time of diagnosis, for example at chest clinics when patients are diagnosed with lung cancer. The role of the specialist nurse in relation to providing support, information and resources is often not clear cut. Macmillan nurses provide advice to carers, patients and professionals about a range of cancer related issues such as symptom control and obtaining small grants to purchase essential equipment. They are also able to provide help with the provision of night sitting services in some areas of the country. Hunt's (1991a) research into the role of symptom control nurses who specialised in the care of the dying patents, suggested that one of the key strategies used by these nurses was to get to know the family and the patient through talk and informal means.

The health and well-being of the primary caregivers

The primary caregiver is invariably the person who bears the majority of the responsibility for caring, even though they may not always be the person with direct physical contact with the patient, although in practice this is unusual. Most patients with a long term chronic condition for example MND, MS, and some cancers, at some point in their lives are likely to have spent time in hospital, even if it was only at the time of diagnosis. In some cases the experience may not always have been a good one and may play a part in the development of a certain amount of reluctance to return. Having said this, others find the hospital experience a positive one and the staff very helpful; in particular when the patient is admitted for respite care and it is well-known to the patient and staff that the patient will return home after a short stay. Often close family members will willingly take up the obligation of caring for each other during illness and in some cases do an exceptionally good job. This is often not unacknowledged by 'the professionals' who, in certain circumstances see the patient only when the carer has become physically/mentally exhausted and incapable of continuing the care of the patient's medical condition, resulting in their admission to hospital. Sykes' (1992) study found that although family members appreciated the care provided by nurses, poor communication and badly organised care was often cited as an area for improvement. The patient's admission may also involve a sense of guilt and despair on the carers' behalf since it is they who, up until now have borne the brunt of the responsibility of the care. As a result of palliation often beginning earlier in the patient's disease process, its duration from onset of terminal care to death can exceed many months and even years. This can place tremendous pressure on carers who may, in some cases, feel able to cope with their loved one's illness, if it is limited to a period of time they can cope with. In some cases of Alzheimer's disease, where the patient's social identity is lost and their slow deterioration continues for many years, the carer can become worn out and even require professional help themselves. In other cases, the care of the patient with cancer, MS or MND can become a very heavy burden which the carer cannot cope with and eventually their loved one has to be hospitalised and eventually dies in the hospital or hospice, despite the original intention to die at home. This can be a major source of upset and guilt, causing in some cases problems with the patient's adaptation to their new surroundings.

Support for lay carers

Patients dying at home are often cared for by a number of carers, although nurses and others often identify a primary care provider who takes key responsibility. In many areas around the country there are organisations set up to specifically support lay carers of patients with a wide range of needs, not just those who are dying. One example is the nationwide crossroads care scheme who assist carers with physical and psychological support.

There are however a wide range of carer schemes set up with some local government assistance to provide people with the essential help required to cope with a disabled, chronically sick or dying relative or friend. Such centres are manned by paid workers and volunteers who provide practical and psychosocial help in most major towns and cities. One of their primary functions is to provide information and advice to carers on a range of topics including how to get financial assistance and how to utilise Social Services. In many carer centres there is a local resource room or library with staff available to help carers obtain up to date information, often using computer assisted programs to gain access to support services. Some carers require financial help with the cost of caring and help is available for visiting patients when they are in hospital, as well as advice on obtaining attendance allowance. Many carer schemes provide help with access to other existing care agencies such as support groups.

Carers providing care to dying patients have many needs; some can take the form of a need for counselling, others require more practical help with holidays and respite care. Some carers want a listening ear and someone with the necessary time, to share the burden of care within a environment in which they can relax and receive empathic and sympathetic responses. In some cases carers can be provided with a designated key worker who will support and help them on an individual basis. In other cases, carers can sit in with small support groups to discuss and share their worries and concerns with those who may have similar difficulties. Many areas operate 'drop in centres' and carers' forums where groups of carers can have a say in both current and future developments. For further information about care schemes see the Useful contacts section on page 201.

District nurses also provide a post-bereavement visit usually carried out by the named community nurses in order to provide support after death. Families, particularly those where the main care provider lives alone after the death, often feel very isolated after the death of a loved one at home. The feeling of loneliness can often be compounded by the fact that so much care has been put into the terminal phase of the patient's illness. District nurses often place great value on the bereavement or 'after death' visit:

> It has proved very effective for the main carer who doesn't feel as though they have been dropped like a hot brick.

The provision of 'after death' support, both from institutional staff and community nurses is a very debatable issue. Many community nurses feel that to suddenly stop visiting the family lacks respect, although it is often difficult to plan and implement a visit to discuss the dead when the living have so many problems requiring time and attention. Nurses in community and hospital settings find it difficult to find the time to reflect back on the care of the dying person and to frame this within a bereavement context (Costello 1996). What follows, is a more personal account of the care provided to my dying Father in our family home.

Dying at home: a personal perspective

The following description provides an abridged account of my Father's death in 1988 which was published in the *Nursing Times* (Costello 1990). My Father's death and the motivation to write a journal paper about it stemmed from a strong desire to share the experience of his death with others, in particular, nurses like myself, as well as those carers who were perhaps facing the impending death of a loved one and the dilemma of 'should I or shouldn't I care for them at home?' There are many advantages as well as disadvantages in making the decision to care for terminally ill loved ones at home. For many dying people, it represents the place where they feel safe, surrounded by those who love them most. For the carer, it can mean a huge responsibility, with many challenges that they feel they want to take on, but may eventually become overwhelmed by as a result of the emotional issues and practical problems involved in caring for a dying person at home. Figure 8.2 illustrates some of the opportunities to be gained from caring for a dying person at home as well as some of the problems.

Opportunities	Potential problems
Knowing that you are more likely to be with them when they die	Being 'out of your depth' and unable to manage their care effectively
Understanding their personal needs	Feeling overwhelmed and experiencing 'compassion fatigue'
Being able to determine their own care	Experiencing the sense of frustration if hospitalisation is needed
Having intimate knowledge of their wants and desires	Having to carry out intimate personal care
Having time to spend with them	Having little or no time to yourself
Being proactive in planning their care	Feeling tired and exhausted
Gaining self satisfaction that you did everything you could to help them	Having little or no support
Helping to ensure they have a 'good death'	Things go wrong, not achieving good pain and symptom control

Figure 8.2 Dying at home: opportunities and problems

The primary caregiver as a nurse

When my Father was diagnosed with cancer of the rectum requiring surgery, I was full of anxieties. He was 67 years old, lived alone and was still able to vividly recall the experience of my Mother's death 7 years earlier in 1981. As a family, my older brother, three sisters and I were devastated by my Mother's death. She died in hospital 6 weeks after being diagnosed with lung cancer. The experience was very painful and left us with many sad memories. Mum was cared for in a large Nightingale type surgical ward of a general hospital. She developed brain metastases, became confused and was in a great deal of pain and distress for the last weeks of her life.

A number of writers have argued that one of the most prevalent feelings when someone is diagnosed with a life threatening condition is fear (Kubler-Ross 1970, Katz & Sidell 1994, Copp 1999). This fear includes anxiety about the type of death and a series of 'what if?' questions, such as what if I die suddenly?, what if my family are not there?, what if I am in pain? and what if I suffer? In my Mum's case, her fears were that of pain. Her pain generated frustration among the family, particularly in my sister, who as an assertive American, could not understand why a dying woman was only given pain relief every two hours, not as required. I can remember vividly how, beside herself with frustration, my sister accosted a casualty houseman when the ward could not contact the doctor to prescribe more analgesia. Shocked by the inflexibility of the system, she literally dragged the poor junior houseman to Mum's bedside and demanded that he prescribe analgesia, which, after checking with his colleague, he did.

Most people fear their last illness will be painful. Unless care is exceptional, studies suggest that one-fifth of patients dying in hospital endure a distressing degree of physical discomfort for an appreciable proportion of the time.

One of the overarching features of my Father's death, in contrast to my Mother's death, was the extent to which the family had control over the management of his death. Dad was found to have secondary cancer spread following the abdominal-perineal resection which showed that the tumour had anastamosed to his bladder and could not be completely removed. His prognosis was poor. When my wife and I became aware of this, it wasn't so much a decision but an inevitability that, despite having a 3 year old son, we agreed to take care of him at home.

My Mum's death had convinced me that I could not endure a repetition of the experience. When Dad was discharged to us, the district nurses provided the necessary skill and support we needed and a very amiable relationship was soon established between us. One problem was whether Dad ought to know the diagnosis and likely outcome of his operation. As a family, knowing his fears and reactions to the word cancer, we thought it best not to tell him, unless he asked.

The GP and district nurses however were of the opinion that he ought to be told the truth, but agreed to respect our wishes. My own experience is that many patients have a clear idea that they are dying, but do not wish to hurt other people by making them aware that they know this (Costello 2000a). Perhaps my knowledge and experience as a nurse helped to influence the family, as my brother and sisters valued my opinion. I sense that had I not been a nurse, things may have been very different. If my father had been nursed in hospital, it is clear that the issue could have produced conflict between the family and the staff.

There is a view that if a doctor conceals from a patient that he is mortally ill and that patient then fails to put his affairs in order, the doctor is in some way negligent (Hinton 1972). However, many doctors are reluctant to speak of death, as they feel patients do not wish to raise the subject except to get reassurance and the truth is likely to be hurtful. Several months after the operation, as predicted by the consultant, Dad became unable to walk without a good deal of pain. We moved his bed into the front room and got him a wheelchair. The psychological implications of being wheelchair-bound, combined with increased pain, caused him some distress.

Distress is a subjective symptom and something many people find difficult to define or measure accurately. Many patients nursed in hospital in the terminal phase of illness suffer pain with associated psychological discomfort and are said to be in distress. The distress of the hospital patient is often attributable not only to the pain, but to the way the person feels about the environment.

Communication

Poor communication can cause more suffering than many of the symptoms of the terminal disease. A study of patients' experience of pain in hospital has shown that the complaints of pain were influenced in a significant way by the nature of the relationship the patient had with the nursing staff. More recent studies suggest that the attitude of staff towards the severely ill patient is important in determining his psychosocial status.

As a family we talked about the end many times and discussed the various scenarios that could confront us. My biggest fear was of getting up in the morning and finding Dad dead on the floor. I often did find him on the floor, because he insisted on trying to get out of bed as soon as he woke up, despite being unable to stand. It had become something of an obsession and it drove my wife and I mad with concern and frustration.

Towards the end, pneumonia developed. We discussed with the doctor the possibility of not actively treating the pneumonia. He had a chat with Dad and learnt that he was anxious to see his daughter who was flying from the US and was due to arrive the next week. On the basis that antibiotics would help him and extend his life, the doctor prescribed a 48-hour course of penicillin. After that we agreed to let nature take its course.

My sister arrived 2 days later and all the family were home. We had 19 for dinner that night and the whole weekend was a special occasion. On the Saturday evening Dad lay in bed in the front room, we played Trivial Pursuits and he answered the question 'Who was the heavyweight boxing champion between 1936 and 1939?' He got the answer right – Joe Louis.

One problem we had encountered during my Mother's terminal phase was not being able to visit her as a whole family. The presence of family members is as important to the patient dying in hospital as it is to the person who dies at home. Although the relatives of dying patients are made to feel very welcome in hospital wards and visiting rules are relaxed, it does cause problems for nursing staff who have to cope with large numbers of often distressed people. Facilities provided for them to spend time being 'around' the patient without actually sitting by the bedside, are often inadequate.

During his last weekend, Dad did not seem to be in any pain, despite being weak and tired. We were using morphine sulphate elixir 30 mg and co-codamol for pain relief. The district nurses came every morning and we carried out the necessary nursing care in the evening. The routine we developed was flexible; sometimes the district nurses would call in at lunchtime just to see how things were. We were offered more nursing support than we needed and because of the availability of people, we chose to do things our own way and thankfully were supported in this.

I had feared the children would be upset by Dad's illness, but in fact the adults were more affected by the situation. The children were a source of stimulation and encouraged us all to organise ourselves and not to sit around waiting for the inevitable. It created a very strong bond between us and in a sense, the children 'normalised' the situation, which was rapidly looking very bleak for my Father.

End of life

Dad deteriorated slowly. His breathing was shallow, but he tolerated fluids and he was conscious and able to express his wishes most of the time. There was always someone with him during the day, and at night my brother and I took it in turns to sleep on the sofa in the same room, give him drinks and make him comfortable. On Tuesday morning the district nurses came at their usual time, while they were changing his pyjama top his breathing pattern worsened, with Cheyne-Stokes respirations and within minutes he died.

The 'end' occurred quickly. Dad had not been in any discomfort or distress. I appreciate that the experience of people dying at home is different from that of hospital patients. I was an experienced nurse and my wife an experienced occupational therapist, which made a tremendous difference, as we were able to deal with his often demanding physical needs. In the absence of immediately available, skilled professional care, physical discomfort may not be dealt with at once in the home and many patients can and do suffer distress, because of the inability of carers to recognise the symptoms. Home care is not always enough to cope properly with the cleaning and dressing of open sores and ulcers, which may then become painful.

On reflection it seems to me that we were in a position to give my Father a tremendous amount of freedom during the latter part of his life. We were able to take him to the pub, allow him to smoke when he wished, but above all we were able to provide him with immediate access to all those people who had meant so much to him during his life. I had been a nurse 10 years and cared for many dying patients. When I reflect on the death of my father – at home, in peace – I can safely say I have experienced what can only be described as a 'good' death.

Reflections on death at home

It is doubtful whether such a dignified death would have been possible if I had not been a nurse and had not had the support of a large, caring family. Unless hospitals are able to change the emphasis on institutional needs to individual needs, then it will always be extremely difficult for somebody to die in a truly patient-centred way. Patients and their families in hospital need private time to talk, cry and to share physical closeness. Although this is possible even in a busy general hospital ward, my experience is that it is often not enough to meet the needs of the dying person and their family.

In my Father's case, being at home meant that he felt safe, he knew and trusted the people around him. In contrast there is very little time to get to know patients in hospital and organisational constraints leave little opportunity for nurses to get to know the patients' real needs. In many instances after death, the family find themselves ushered away from the scene as the practicalities of dealing with the body are organised. There is therefore little time to begin the process of bereavement.

Because Dad died among his family, in an environment he knew and understood, it helped us to come to terms with his death. We did not feel alienated from him and after his death, he lay in the front room and we each had time to go and say or do what we wanted without feeling constrained by ward handovers, doctors' availability and the need for the bed to be vacated.

My Mother's illness in hospital, the experience of visiting someone in pain daily, is a vivid memory that has diminished in intensity. I wish we had had the opportunity when Mum died, to sit down and discuss in an informed way, how our family may have coped with the death. On reflection, the decision to admit her to hospital was made without consultation, and before we knew where we were, she was in hospital dying and we were trying to brace ourselves for the impending event.

Based on my personal experience it seems that when a patient is terminally ill, it would be useful, I feel, to have a case conference where the doctor, the patient's relatives and/or the patient and community nurses can sit and discuss the most dignified way in which the person can spend his or her last days. Too often, hospital staff take control, excluding the family from caregiving. Sometimes this can be a relief for the relatives. Deciding what people want and how to facilitate their wishes is a skill based on knowledge, experience and sensitivity, which need to be extended towards the family and the patient. My experience of having my Father die with us at home was sad but very rewarding. It helped the family come to terms with the loss because, with the appropriate support of doctors and nurses, we felt truly involved in the provision of care and it helped us to cope with the sorrow, which often accompanies the death of a loved one. When I look back now on the death of my parents, my Mother's death was traumatic because it seemed so sudden and we never seemed to have any control over events at the time. I recall it being a time of anxiety and in many ways it could be categorised as a 'bad death' in the sense that there was a lot of anger, frustration and a range of negative emotions such as guilt and denial. Moreover there was a sense of impotence and a sense of not being able to have any influence over what seemed like a nightmare taking place before us.

In contrast, my Father's death could be seen as a 'good death' in the sense that we were prepared for and had talked about his death. We felt that he knew what was going to happen. We also experienced a great sense of unity and togetherness about what was going on. We were very much in control and the professional staff involved helped and supported us to maintain this. It appears, looking back, that this is what their role was. At all times we felt involved, in all the decisions made and the initiation of events such as changes in medication and the timing of interventions. This was so important to us at the time. The skills that were used by the professionals were the human ones of discretion, sensitivity and the need to help us maintain dignity and peace. The death of my parents taught my family many things. Most of all I learnt that the death of a loved one does not have to be full of sadness and despair but can, with the right help, be an opportunity for personal growth.

Problems caring for dying people at home

Bos (2003) discusses the problem of the patient not wanting to go into hospital despite the professional advice. In describing a professional encounter with a dehydrated patient who refuses to go into hospital against the GP's advice, she points out that essentially, it is important that wherever possible the patient's wishes are acknowledged and acted upon. The patient she described had not eaten for days and was dehydrated. After making an action plan with a community nurse colleague, Bos manages to stabilise the patient and after 5 days a niece visits and insists her uncle be admitted to hospital. Bos points out that she is helping her uncle to die which he does a few days later. His death was peaceful and he seemed happy. This vignette raises two important issues. First, the need for patient autonomy and the desire to have their last wishes met. Second, there is also the carer's autonomy. In community settings nurses are often faced with difficult decisions about whether patients should die at home or go to hospital. In some cases the patient wants to be at home but recognises that there may not be sufficient resources to care for them at home. This is a major issue and requires careful consideration. Having several family members involved does not always make the decision making any easier. All too often the family consider the needs of the dying person and agonise over what they want and what can be provided. Hospital care offers a secure safe solution sometimes as a compromise between the desires of the patient, and the ability of the family to provide effective care. In some cases emergencies may take place when caring for a patient at home, such as a cardiac arrest or a bout of uncontrollable pain. When situations like this take place, it is important to seek help. This can take the form of a visit from the GP, community/Macmillan nurses or the emergency services. In some cases the patient is taken to hospital for acute treatment. These problems are often not foreseeable and may occur at any time of the day or night. Good communication between the primary care staff and planning and preparation for such events can help to alleviate some of the tension and anxiety that is part of the many difficulties encountered when a person is dying at home.

For many people caring for the dying at home is hard work and often lonely, especially if the dying person is unable to communicate.

Axelsson & Sjoden (1998) point out that many carers feel unsure about leaving the dying person and so tend to stay at home rather than ask others to 'take over' to enable them to go out for a walk or to do some shopping. When my Father was dying, the family arranged for numerous people including friends to 'Dad sit' to enable my wife and I to go out or to take Dad to the pub. One evening we had booked seats to go the theatre. My brother was late getting to the house and before we left we gave Dad his usual morphine and left in a hurry as soon as my brother arrived. When we returned my Dad was in a deep sleep and my brother explained that he had also given dad his morphine and a couple of glasses of Guinness! Dad slept well that night and woke next day stating he had the best night's sleep for a long time!

Summary

This chapter has examined the possibilities as well as some of the problems and challenges involved in caring for a dying person at home. I have illustrated the chapter with a personal perspective in order to highlight the practical and emotional issues that face the primary caregivers. I would stress that my experiences are unique in a number of ways. First, as a registered nurse with an occupational therapist as a wife, our task was easier than most. My family was large and we had many friends who, like us, were young, knowledgeable, physically fit and aware of some of the problems encountered with dying people. These things make a difference when caring for a dying person at home. Above all we had the support of an excellent primary care team. The support from others and the resources of a professional team are essential ingredients for success. It has been over a decade since Dad died. The care for dying patients in the community has improved and progressed. Palliative care at home is rapidly developing and there is a wide range of services available to support carers who decide to adopt the role of primary care provider. The extension of palliative care in the home opens up a whole area in which professionals and lay carers can work together. One of the key issues, which appears to be a feature of effective palliative care in any setting is good communication and openness about expectations of care. I would endorse this view from the literature and add that teamwork between professionals and lay care providers is one of the most important issues arising from the care of dying people in their own home.

Further reading

Cobb M. (2001) *The dying soul: spiritual care at the end of life.* OU Books, Buckingham.

This is one of the few books about spirituality written in clear understandable terms that seeks to make sense of life and death issues. Based on the author's experience of numerous people, the book looks at spirituality from the dying person's perspective, but also looks at those who provide spiritual care at the end of life.

Department of Social Security (2000) *A guide to benefits.* DSS Communications. Belmont Press, Leeds.

This free small booklet available from Social Security offices provides details of all benefits payable to people who have difficulty in their activities of daily living and those who are disabled and terminally ill, adults and children. It also provides advice to families on low incomes and gives information about how to claim and what to do if you find yourself in financial difficulty as a result of ill health.

Department of Social Security (2000a) *What to do after a death in England and Wales.* DSS Communications. Belmont Press, Leeds.

This is government guide available free from the benefits agency which explains what must be carried out when a death takes place in a range of contexts from hospital to abroad. It also provides a wealth of information about arranging a funeral and the help that is available for bereaved people.

Hinton J. (1972) *Dying.* Penguin Books, London.

This is one of the most interesting paperback books on death and dying and is a true classic. Written by a GP, this book looks at dying from a very sensitive perspective and is comprehensive, scholarly and humane without being sentimental. The book is very readable and one of the 'must read' texts about death and dying for those seriously interested in caring for dying people.

Thomas K. (2003) *Caring for the dying at home: companions on the journey.* Radcliffe Medical Press, Abingdon.

This is an extremely useful and well-written book based on the author's personal and professional experiences as a GP and a regional advisor to Macmillan Cancer Relief. The underlying philosophy of the book is a very humane one as the author points out that dying is important to all of us, irrespective of where we die, although when people die at home they and their care providers need encouragement and support along the journey. This book sets out the author's model for a good death at home known as the Gold Standard Framework (GSF), which is a practical tool for helping people to coordinate and communicate ways of managing death at home to maximise the dying person's experience and support the carer at all times. It is a useful book for professional and lay carers although it is largely focused on professional care providers.

9 Caring for the dying in post-modern society

Introduction

Advances in medical technology and health care have demonstrated significant improvements in disease detection and treatment, particularly at the 'cutting edge' of genetic screening and most significantly the ability to preserve the life of premature babies from as young as 20 weeks' gestation. Despite these important innovations, many critics of the health care system point towards the lack of quality in the care of dying people within NHS establishments, as discussed in detail in Chapters 1 and 2. Many of the criticisms resonate with more general problems associated with and widely published in the literature. These relate to poor communication, a lack of dignity and the inability of health care workers to individualise the care of the dying person.

The purpose of the final chapter is to reflect on previous discussions concerning nursing care at the end of life and to contextualise death and dying in post-modern society. This includes a consideration of post-modernist values and ideas about society and the way in which social control is maintained. It also includes and examines current debates about the way in which death and dying has become medicalised and professionalised by the dominant professional groups in our society. The chapter also looks at the role of modern nursing care for dying people, in particular the role of nurses in relation to good and bad death scenarios and the bereavement support given to families who are facing impending death.

Death in a post-modern world

Death is much more than an outcome of dying and is the single most important social factor of human existence. For the majority of people, the context in which death takes place has a significant effect, not only on the social process of dying but also because of its influence on shaping societal and individual attitudes about mortality. Death raises many profound social and cultural issues about its importance to society and the value placed upon life. In the past, western society's attitude towards death and dying was characterised by denial and avoidance, as many researchers have testified (Feifel 1959, Gorer 1987, Littlewood 1992, Kastenbaum 1996). More recently, writers have began to question the notion that we are a death denying society. In particular the work of Tony Walter (1994) highlights what he refers to as a '*revival of death*', in which he points out that people are becoming increasingly more interested in the process of dying, and the management or disposal of the body after death. It may be argued that Walter and others are highlighting a major change in attitude towards death and dying, which reflects post-modern thinking and values about a topic traditionally referred to as a taboo subject. Contemporary writing on death and dying challenges social researchers to develop an understanding of what death means and to consider its influence on social organisation in a post-modern context. It is also useful to consider how ideas about social organisation have changed past and current influences on social development.

Modernity

Modernity in a chronological sense refers to the historical period beginning with the age of enlightenment around the end of the 18th century characterised by the secularisation of societies and the rise of scientific and philosophical rationalisation (Fox 1993). Foucault (1970) identifies this period with the birth of the modern scientific disciplines of economics, biology and languages. Modernism is characterised by a commitment to truth and rationality with knowledge being embedded in scientific truth giving rise to the birth of humanism, with humans being the focus of knowledge and human discourse.

The shift from modernity to post-modernism is less to do with chronology and more to do with a paradigm shift in thinking from religious to the secular. In terms of post-modernist thinking, many writers argue that what has been recognised as reality has been replaced by simulation, rationality by multivocality and monolithic organisation by fragmentation (Fox 1993). More recently Grbich (2003) points out that post-modernism reflects an eclectic approach indicating that human society is constituted in language and that through a series of discourses based on language, reconstruction with social structures in post-modernist society becomes mediated through talk and social constructions of reality (Kellner 1988, Flax 1990, Bauman 1992 and Lemert 1992). In terms of nursing, reconstruction is the move from the traditional caring model with the notion of presence (the ability to claim unmediated knowledge) (Watson 1999:22). As Watson (1999:85) points out:

> The modern lens of nursing, medicine, western science and the western world refracted out the feminine principle from nursing and humankind.

Modernity and post-modernity are interwoven in a transformative process and by their very nature almost impossible to define. Post-modernism attempts to incorporate aspects of modernity to recognise the socially constructed nature of the world. Grbich (2003:22) points out that post-modernism characterised by the search for reality is qualified by a recognition that the tools, language and processes of discovery are socially and culturally constructed and require further examination. Many post-modern texts indicate that post-modernism is about the capacity for dialogue with other contextual and temporal influences and that borders to the development of reality are also constructions that can be crossed, incorporated or reconstructed.

Post-modernism and health care

In a post-modern society the organisation of health care in general and the management of death in particular is seen to have undergone considerable change as a result of responses made to changing social patterns and the development of a new culture of grief (Walter 1999). Scrutiny appears to be placed on the care provided to dying patients. In hospital it is argued that as much as 50% of all care and treatment is palliative, with a significant shift in the provision of palliative care from institutions to the community context (Biswas 1993). In particular, the emergence of palliative care as a medical speciality and the structural changes in health care provision (including financial constraints) has meant that palliative care is being provided more outside of mainstream NHS hospitals. This may pose a problem for importing recognised quality approaches to care such as Integrated Care Pathways and HBSPCTs. These, as discussed in Chapter 5, are seen as the gold standard of palliative care. However they may not always be the right approach in all contexts (Leese 2002). An example of the difficulties of implementing ICPs in the community is the lack of involvement of the carer or 'consumer' in care pathways within a context where the professional cannot always adopt the type of high profile enjoyed in institutional contexts.

In answer to the questions raised in Chapters 1 and 2 regarding the problems with terminal care in hospitals, it is important to consider that as institutions, they are, as Revans (1974) points out, '*cradled in anxiety*'. Revans' argument is based on the observation that hospitals are constantly trying to construct a reality pivoted on conflict between professional groups, largely doctors and nurses and other interested parties such as administrators. Another consideration is the discrepancy between the needs of the organisation, which are often placed before those of the patient (Mackay 1993). A major problem with hospital care highlighted in Chapter 3, is the way in which rules, routines and organisational needs permeated and controlled hospital life. It is recognised that most institutions involve rule making and conformity to the goals of the organisation (Douglas 1977). Living and dying in hospital it has been argued, poses a problem for patients in being able to express their individual needs, despite the rhetoric that professional nursing is all about individualised care (Mackay 1989). Paradoxically, as the evidence suggests, there is little individuality in relation to death and dying in hospital (Lawler 1991). There are also a number of hurdles to be overcome such as communicating effectively and becoming cognisant of the role requirements of the patient or 'how to play the game' (Goffman 1968). Goffman (1968) points out that people in institutions have a number of responsibilities to enable their stay to become free from organisational friction. The reality of dying in hospital, as Chapter 5 points out, is that many patients are often not told the truth about their medical condition and open disclosure of information about the patient is a problematic issue for many doctors and nurses caring for dying patients.

Specialist care

Ways of improving care in hospitals (discussed in Chapter 5) included HBSPCTs. These teams utilise the services of a small number of specialist nurses and doctors working in hospital. Evidence from a survey of Macmillan post holders in the UK suggests that whilst being effective in their role of helping others to improve services, the practice support needs of these individuals go unrecognised (Booth et al 2003). It is also perhaps interesting to note that the development of HBSPC teams has the potential to threaten the cohesion of multi-disciplinary team working of hospital based staff (Jack et al 2002). The development of HBSPC teams, and the difficulties these small and often isolated teams have experienced highlights the problem that it is often not the structure or function of a group of specialists that creates tensions, but the context in which they operate. The problems appear to emanate from within the environment in which nurses operate as a result of the organisational constraints they encounter. Paradoxically nurses are encouraged to engage in multi-disciplinary working, although the source of much conflict resides within such relationships. It is also worth considering the potential threat posed by HBSPCTs in relation to de-skilling the generalist nurse (Jack et al 2002).

More recently, a systematic review of the literature relating to Hospital Based Specialist Palliative Care Teams carried out by Higginson et al (2002) suggests that they do offer benefits in terms of providing staff with advice and education about pain and symptom control. These findings however should be interpreted cautiously since there is little evidence that patient care is directly affected by such teams who often have no direct link to dying patients. Support from specialist teams does not take into account the organisational culture of the hospital and is thus 'culturally sterile'. One of the positive impacts of HBSPCTs is to change the referral patterns, which traditionally existed when patients were being discharged from hospital. Where such teams exist in hospitals they may therefore function as a 'filter', whereby patients with potential problems prior to discharge can be identified and referred to other specialist services such as community Macmillan nurses.

Hospices: the ideal place to die?

Despite home being the preferred place of death for most people, the vast majority are admitted into institutional care towards the end of life and most die in hospital as the early part of the book described. In post-modern society, outside the home, the ideal place for dying patients appears to be the hospice, which, despite only admitting a minority of patients, occupies the 'blue chip standard' in relation to palliative and terminal care. Hospices clearly emerge in the literature and in practice as specialist centres of care for patients with cancer and non-cancer conditions, although patients with the former disease are more likely to secure access to most hospices (Seale & Kelly 1997). In terms of post-modern dying, hospices offer a homely and welcoming context in which to die. The patient, family and friends are encouraged to share the opulent facilities and to spend time with their loved ones. For the patient, the individuality of care within a secure and well-resourced environment offers the peace and security rarely found in NHS hospitals (Dunphy & Amesbury 1990). Patient centred care in a hospice focuses on the notion of holism, which takes into account not only medical needs but cultural, social and spiritual dimensions. Hospices however are not without their problems and challenges, as a number of writers have identified (Kastenbaum 1982, Russ 1989, Miller 1992, Logue 1994).

Hospice care with its hotel-like environment described as a 'health farm for the dying' is more a 'theme park for the terminally ill' with personalised service, snoozelums, hydrotherapy pools, massage, complementary therapies and serene places for worship and tranquillity (Clark 2002a). For the very small number of patients who die there, despite the luxury, hospices still represent institutional care. Compared with hospitals and their impersonal and sometimes woeful detachment from the patient, hospices are seen as centres of excellence. There is however evidence that despite their hallowed status, hospice care can become routinised (Field & James 1993), elitist (Douglas 1992), and difficult to gain access to (Clark & Seymour 1999).

The limits of palliative care

Chapter 4 provided an account of hospice care in a small modern hospice contrasting the relative luxury of the hospice setting with the impersonal care of hospitals described in earlier chapters. One of the primary problems identified with hospice care is its limited access to patients with non-malignant conditions such as Alzheimer's disease, Multiple Sclerosis and Motor Neurone Disease which perhaps give rise to criticisms that hospice care is limited to a privileged few who suffer mainly from cancer (Seale 1991). Kastenbaum (1982) highlights what he calls '*healthy dying*' in relation to the American way of managing death – the notion that dying should be exalting and fulfilling. He explains that this was a major fantasy of the public at large fostered mainly by the hospice movement. Limitations of hospice care have been identified by a number of other writers who point out that hospices tend to select the 'best patients' and those with very unmanageable symptoms are rarely encountered (Logue 1994). Others point out that hospices are unable to provide the type of pain control discussed by Saunders (1988) without rendering the patient unconscious (Battin 1989). Clark & Seymour (1999) point out that in the UK, some of the social care provided by hospices can be obtained externally by non-specialist care providers at much less cost. For some patients, hospices, like visits from Macmillan nurses, may 'conjure up' an image of dying and represent the road towards death. This may be because people in general equate hospices and Macmillan nurses with death, causing some to refuse the invitation for Macmillan nurse involvement in care. Despite the anecdotal evidence of patients being admitted to hospital and dying unexpectedly, to a limited extent, the same could be said of hospice care (particularly in the past). More recently hospices have made many advances in converting their image from a place of death to one focusing on 'fine tuning' of symptoms (Wilkinson & Mula 2003). In the last decade, lengths of stay in hospices for patients whose conditions remain stable or improve, have reduced and in many modern hospices patients are admitted for shorter periods to the point where arrangements for returning home are made on the day of admission (Eve & Smith 1996).

The medicalisation of death and dying

The medicalisation of death has been a recurrent topic of debate within palliative care for many years since the onus for implementing terminal care shifted from the family to professional groups. Advances in medical science and technology have resulted in an increasing prolongation of life for many patients with cancer and non-cancer conditions, often initiating a protracted period of illness requiring palliative care. Although seen by many as an attempt to improve the care of the dying, the emergence of palliative medicine and nursing care as a specialty area in the 1980s may also be seen as part of the medicalisation of death. Historically, just as death and dying became taboo subjects, today, the prevention and control of death in post-modern society, has become a primary cultural value in many westernised countries. A number of writers have questioned the extent to which palliative care has encouraged this shift towards professionals taking over this traditional family role (Field 1994, Seymour 1999). Traditional death, which closely involved families giving the locus of control to the dying person, has conceptually and practically ceased to exist in post-modern society. This may be due to several factors; increased incidence of institutionalised deaths, social demographic changes and changing societal attitudes towards death in general. Berger & Luckman (1991 (originally 1967: 119) remark that:

> Needless to elaborate, death also posits the most terrifying threat to the taken-for-granted realities of everyday life. The integration of death within the reality of social existence is, therefore, of the greatest importance for any institutional order.

In palliative care contexts it may be argued that the push towards controlling the symptoms of cancer and non-cancer conditions gives rise to what Saunders' (1988) called *total pain control* (whereby the patient becomes free from their distressing problems).

In itself this may be seen as evidence of the medicalisation of death and dying.

Medicalisation: the end of death?

Medical domination of health care has become a major feature of post-modern life in the last decade. Sociologists and philosophers having debated its influence on our daily lives, recognise that the primary goal of medicine is to prevent and control death, which is seen both as a threat and a failure (Kearl 1989, Illich 1990). Seymour (1999) points out that the medicalisation thesis forms part of wider moves within society to become free from medical intervention and return to more natural forms of death and dying. Medical science however may be seen as having the ability to control or cure death. Illich's (1990) thesis, that consumer society has become conditioned by medicine to believe that all its ills are potentially curable, is under-pinned by the pervasive ideology that there is a cure for every ill including old age, impotence and infertility. Over the years, the role of modern medicine in relation to terminal care has interested many sociologists and physicians, who have expressed concern about its role in transforming patterns of death and dying (Ahmedzai 1993, Clark 1993, Field 1994, Walter 1994). Historically, as the literature reflects, dying was a highly personalised social activity mainly involving the family and others, who utilised a series of symbolic, practical and culturally prescribed leave-taking rituals, to acknowledge the deceased's departure from the material world. The medicalisation of death and dying has made private, what was once a public social event and in so-doing, has de-personalised it as an event that takes place in institutions such as hospitals and hospices surrounded by professionals, rather than at home surrounded by the family. McNamara et al (1994) discuss the increasing institutionalisation of hospice care arguing that it may pose a threat to the founding ideals of the hospice movement. The emergence of hospices as centres of excellence together with the increasing contribution of biomedical science to palliative care in terms of chemical methods of controlling symptoms, have formed a symbiosis whereby hospice care is an icon of palliative care. It may be argued that hospices have lost sight of their 'grass roots' and links with palliative care principles encapsulated in the phrase 'to cure sometimes but to care always'.

Good deaths in hospital and hospice settings

Chapter 5 looked critically at hospital care, highlighting the numerous problems associated with the provision of high quality care within a culture where power struggles between nurses and doctors existed and where the predominant ethos was patient control. Within this context health care staff struggled to meet the challenges involved in providing patients with a 'good death'. The concept of the good death is often associated with euthanasia, although from a practical perspective, nurses caring for the dying describe good deaths as powerful experiences revealing rich insights into the way death is managed. As Hopkinson (2002) and others have pointed out, the history of hospital deaths is a history of the search for the traditional 'good death'. Definitions of the good death vary although in general terms they are often described in terms of being comfortable and peaceful, as well as involving high levels of dignity and personal autonomy. Above all, many describe the good death as being free from distress and suffering (McNamara et al 1994, Field & Cassel 1997, Lynch & Abrahm 2002). The notion of a good death according to Ten Have (2003), has its own ideology promoted largely by the hospice movement in general and by palliative care practitioners in particular. The aim of traditional palliative care, it may be argued is the promotion of a good death although for a number of reasons, within many institutions, the good death may be neither feasible nor desirable.

Death within western society is often viewed in a personal individualised way. Dying is personal, with people encouraged to choose their own approach to dying (Kearl 1989, Walter 1994). In order to accurately assess interpretations of good death we need to incorporate the symbolic meanings associated with death and avoid uncritically adopting the notion of ideal type death scenarios such as home deaths as the best form of death. In many cases a death at home where the carer is unprepared and unable to provide the necessary care can be a very onerous situation, more commonly found in a hospital. Nurses in hospice settings often want patients to have the type of death that excludes distress, limited suffering and stress to both the patient and themselves (Costello & Horne 2003). Evidence suggests that nurses' perceptions of good and bad deaths in hospital focus much on the way organisational issues are structured and include issues such as whether the death was well managed, if the patient was aware that they were dying and the level of preparation made for death by nurses and patients (Kellehear 1992). My hospital-based research (Costello 2000) highlighted the need for a much broader analysis of the organisational/structural constraints within health care systems, particularly in relation to the way in which care for older people was organised and implemented. Good death scenarios according to Kellehear (1992:31) are closely associated with the ability of the person to prepare for death. In institutional terms one of the key issues to emerge from the literature was the lack of preparation for death as well as the poor quality of communication about end of life issues in general. This view is supported by others who also reported that dissatisfaction with nursing care in hospital at the end of life was associated with lack of information about the dying process (Rogers et al 2000). Indications from this research suggests that if a palliative care approach had been taken, much of the frustration about death could have been alleviated especially by patients whose deaths were anticipated. Ackroyd (1993) and others point out that deaths that are well managed can bring satisfaction for nurses and patients. One of the respondents in this study pointed out that:

> So long as they don't just die in a corner with nobody taking any notice. If you are able to think to yourself, such a body is likely to die in the next day or two, and to make sure that they get the attention they need, you get some satisfaction from a job well done.

Other writers have expressed the view that a good death in hospital is difficult to achieve, citing the fact that many patients may die alone or in pain (Field 1984). The importance of not dying alone is considered important by many nurses who also support the point made by Kellehear's (1992) research that control over the events at the end of life and preparation are key issues in the achievement of a good death.

Bad deaths

In contrast to many writers views on the good death, my personal and professional experience has been that death can be a very negative experience and as a nurse I have experienced what many refer to as 'bad' deaths. The latter term is often used to refer to situations in which the dying process at the end of life and the death itself was poorly managed, unexpected and caused stress to the patient/family and the staff involved. These contrast with the good death experience and involve a lack of preparation, uncontrolled pain and various other symptoms, together with poor communication. Bad deaths may exist as both individual experiences, as well as organisational bad deaths whereby nurses and doctors collectively feel that the death was poorly managed (Costello 2000). Bad death scenarios can result in staff feeling guilty because of their inability to exert control over the death, as well as creating negative memories of the event for the family. In relation to my hospital research, many nurses recalled instances where the death was unexpected and lacked control. One ward sister recalled how a patient died whilst being given a bath. Despite her best efforts and following futile attempts at resuscitation, the patient died in the bathroom. In order to limit distress to other patients, the nurse placed an oxygen mask on the deceased patient, called the porters to fetch a trolley and transferred the patient out of the ward informing other patients that their fellow patient was being taken to the Intensive Care Unit because she 'took a turn for the worst' whilst having a bath. Goffman (1968) refers to situations like this as *'flaws in the performance'* and points out that hospital staff try to keep secret events that go wrong and blemish the professional image. In other instances staff recalled deaths where the patient died suddenly with no time to prepare the family for the bad news. This can involve nurses making phone calls to relatives, not disclosing to them that the patient had died informing them instead of the need to come to the hospital because the patient's condition had become critical. This beneficent lie is common to many nurses and relatives who may confront the nurse by requesting the truth! In other instances of bad deaths, patients may die slowly and in pain with nurses being unable to control their distressing symptoms.

Bad organisational deaths

Bad deaths in organisational terms are those that occur unexpectedly, for example when the patient and family are unprepared for death, perhaps because the possibility of death has not been previously discussed. The discovery on the death certificate that the patient had cancer can cause shock and render the event of death as a negative experience. One nurse was upset by the attitude of the staff when his Father died after having requested that he be allowed to perform last offices on his Father. The nurse in charge responded by pointing out that she felt that his request was inappropriate and 'disgusting'. The son recalled the situation as a bad death scenario because he was unable to have any influence on the dying process and moreover, his grief was compounded by the negative attitude of the nurse. Bad death scenarios involve the negation of expectations, often in direct contrast to good death scenarios. The main characteristics are lack of control over events such as when a cardiac arrest occurs. They may also apply when family members are unhappy about the inappropriate use of CPR and Do Not Resuscitate policy decisions (Costello 2002). In other cases due to a lack of symptoms, death occurs suddenly and leaves the relatives sad and the staff sharing the sense of sadness particularly if the patient was popular. In some cases bad deaths have an adverse effect on both the family and the staff, for example when a patient's pain control is poor and they die in distress with family members observing their last hours of life in distress. An example of a bad death was a patient (Jim) I encountered in my hospital research (Costello 2000) who was not told he was dying. For many months despite asking questions of the staff he was never told that he had lung cancer. The nurses and doctors felt he was confused and was expected to die after a few weeks, although this did not happen. Jim experienced a slow lingering death for many months before dying. His son was unable to visit due to his sadness and inability to tell his father that he was dying (since he had been told the diagnosis by the consultant). After Jim's death, the ward staff called a meeting with the medical staff to express the way they felt about not having told the patient he was dying and how many experienced a sense of guilt about what they felt had been a bad death.

Mission impossible: palliative care at home

One of the most vexing issues surrounding palliative care in general, but death and dying in particular, is to do with meeting the patient's wishes and enabling them to die in the place of their choice (Cartwright 1991, Todd et al 2002). Caring for dying patients at home, as Chapter 8 identified, requires a great deal of effort and support from health professionals. Often caring in professional terms is idealised as an activity carried out by 'experts' trained and educated to become able to fulfil the needs of the patient. In lay terms, caring for a loved one or a friend can be a spontaneous act of kindness or love fostered from a desire to help the other person. Care as Brechin (1998) points out, is available to most people in a variety of contexts. Those with competent families can be cared for in settings suitable to all concerned. For others, without social support networks to help provide the type of care required, institutional care can be provided. Institutional settings however require the patient to adopt a more passive role when making the necessary adaptation needed to fit into their surroundings such as hospices, nursing homes and hospitals. Receiving care at home also requires adjustment, but much less so than the changes patients in hospital are required to make. The latter also requires relatives to abdicate responsibility for care to professionals and the patient is required to conform to the institutional routine. This can be a difficult process especially when the family are not satisfied that the care is of a sufficient standard or where the care is perceived to be below what the patient was receiving at home. Conversely, the patient who is admitted to hospital care because the family were unable to cope, may experience and share a sense of relief and gratitude that their burden has been lifted.

Hospice at home

The provision of hospice care in the patient's home has received a great deal of attention in the last 5 years, largely because of the need to improve standards of care but also as an alternative to institutional care. Hospice at Home programmes strive to ensure that the end of life is as positive an experience as possible for the patient and the family. One example of this is the Cambridge Hospice at Home service which involves providing home care for dying patients in the last 2 weeks of life. The aim of the service is to improve terminal care for patients with a wide range of medical conditions including malignant and non-malignant diseases. Research carried out with the Cambridge scheme by Todd et al (2002) revealed that such care did not seem to make any significant difference to the terminal care of the patient. Neither did it allow more patients to die at home. The death of a patient at home however can allow the principles of palliative care such as the need for cure sometimes and care always, to become a reality. Thomas (2003), discussing the need to holistically assess patients' needs at home, argues for professionals to adopt what she calls '*real listening*' to families' needs and focus in particular on what they want which, it is argued becomes more achievable in the home setting as the professional is in the patient's territory. Thomas advocates the use of 'home packs', which contain feedback sheets for patients who are actively encouraged to participate in the care. These packs are similar to diaries and require the patient or family members to document their views and needs to facilitate listening and help to prioritise future actions.

Reflecting on the death of my Father enables me to consider the value of a home death as well as the many problems associated with enabling death to take place at home. It is important to consider that dying at home should also mean living at home before death and include the care of the family who provide the bulk of the palliative care. It is often these primary carers who need support from health professionals. Palliative care at home challenges professional care providers to consider the issue of having at least two patients to care and provide support to. Palliative care at home is more than an ideal and requires not only resources and positive attitudes, but a commitment to plan, implement and evaluate the care, using the patient's agenda as the central focus. Professional caregivers need to consider that institutional care will always be a secondary preference and if patient autonomy is to become a reality, it is necessary to take steps to ensure that palliative care at home is researched in more detail. The problems need to be evaluated in order to thoroughly reveal strategies for developing effective ways of establishing palliative home care as a major form of nursing and medical intervention for the future.

Bereavement support

The care of dying patients in a variety of contexts often gives rise to concerns from nurses and others about the type of psychological support required by the soon to be bereaved family members. In many hospices risk assessment tools have been developed based largely on the work of Parkes (1972) and others (Parkes et al 1996) which enable staff to identify potential problems which may arise as a result of the patient's death and the circumstances of the bereaved person. In hospital and community situations such tools are rarely used although nurses and doctors express concern about the possible after effects that death may have on surviving family members.

The impending death of a spouse can give rise to a wide range of emotional experiences which take place before death and have become known as anticipatory grief (Rando 1986). Some would argue that there is no such thing as anticipatory grief, pointing out that the various adaptations to loss represent preparation for impending death, pointing out that 'grief is grief' irrespective of its temporality. As research into death and dying has advanced, so has the scope of academic investigation to the extent that it is possible to identify differing grief reactions and the differences between so called normal and abnormal grief reactions (Parkes et al 1996).

The bereavement needs of the family have caused speculation amongst nurses who have attempted to develop hospital bereavement programmes as a way of meeting the needs of family survivors. Many of these initiatives have been developed in the USA and to some extent the UK (Archer 2001). Bereavement support can take many forms from immediate help with practical problems such as registering the death, to invitations from social workers and others to attend memorial events such as the after death day and the 13-month service at St Christopher's (see Parkes et al 1996). In one hospital setting relatives of patients (and ward staff) who have died in the ward in the previous year were invited to return to the hospital for a memorial service conducted by the hospital chaplain in the day room. The aim of the event was to acknowledge the loss in a ritual and public way and demonstrate a form of care continuity after death (Costello 1996). Such events are uncommon, although more nurses are becoming interested in setting up hospital based bereavement programmes. In some areas, such as Accident and Emergency departments, relatives of those who have died as a result of sudden death (such as parents following their child's death), are contacted by telephone and asked if they need any further help. Such support can take many forms including the offer of comfort over the telephone, reassurance and a supportive listener, but can also involve referral to a bereavement counselling agency such as CRUSE, Age Concern or other specialist groups such as the Still Birth and Neonatal Death Society (see Useful contacts section). In many hospices social workers and nurses offer bereavement support as well as trained volunteer counsellors. This is often an integral part of the hospice service, which extends support and palliative care to include bereavement after care. This is an important and at times difficult service to provide, illustrating the holistic approach that has become the symbol of palliative care throughout the world.

The role of the nurse in caring for dying people

One of the central features of both the literature on death and dying as well as my practical experiences of caring for dying people has been the role of the nurse in caring for patients and supporting family members and others before, during and after death. Nurses have the responsibility of ensuring quality of care for the patient and supporting the family during what is clearly a crisis when the patient is diagnosed with a life threatening illness. Nurses have three main roles in relation to terminal care within a wide range of contexts. First, they are part of the culture of care provided to patients and thus need to assess the impact that the setting has on the patient and the family. This includes taking responsibility for ensuring that those admitted into their care feel part of and actively engaged in the care culture. This can be encouraged through patients becoming involved in decision making about issues such as timing of refreshments. Second, nurses need to assess and find ways of engaging with dying patients to ensure that nursing care is appropriate, sensitive to patients' needs and ethically justified. The latter encompasses wide ranging responsibilities to advocate and empower patients, despite the many problems this raises for professional practice (Willard 1996, Mallik 1997). Third, nurses have professional commitments to ensure high standards of care, which include remaining updated on innovations and educated in research and new evidence that seeks to improve care.

Caring as a key concept

The key contextual issue relating to the care of dying people in any context is the quality of the nursing care provided and the perception of that care. Biswas (1993) argues that half the so-called nursing care given to dying patients in hospital is palliative and as such people have started to become more aware of the idea of palliative care. Often nursing care in professional terms is idealised as an activity carried out by 'experts' trained and educated to become able to fulfil the needs of the patient. In lay terms caring for a loved one or a friend is a spontaneous act of kindness or love fostered from a desire to help the other person. Care in this sense, as Brechin (1998) points out is available to most people in a variety of contexts. Nursing care of the dying patient, as Brykczynska (1992) points out, may be seen as both an art and a science asserting that effective nursing care for dying patients involves a wide range of human skills. These include the use of empathy, which does not require the nurse to have had any personal experience of loss. Moreover, nurses need to rely on their level of sensitivity and common understanding of life and life's events in order to become effective in providing humanistic care at the end of life. The social structures in the residential settings (Chapters 6 and 7) highlighted the key role of care staff in the provision of terminal care. My observations lead me to conclude that there is a need for more education and training of this group particularly relating to palliative care provision. There is however some uncertainty about what to do for terminally ill residents, which perhaps can be addressed by greater involvement of residents or their relatives in care practices. This may reduce the dependency of the resident as well as empower those relatives who wish to become involved to make proxy decisions on behalf of their loved ones. Many of the caring skills required in all areas of nursing referred to by Brykczynska (1992) as *the five Cs (commitment, competence, confidence, conscience and compassion)* are essential when caring for dying patients irrespective of the context.

Organisational issues

Nursing care of the dying patient is effective if the nurse is able to assess not only the patient but also become aware of the contextual problems that impinge on the provision of high quality care. This includes paying attention to organisational issues such as the making of DNR orders and the need for transparency in developing end of life care plans. Importantly nurses need to ensure that doctors clearly prescribe appropriate medication, ensuring that anticipated problems associated with pain and other symptoms are prepared for, such as break through pain and medication administration quickly using the most appropriate route. Nurses need also to be vigilant about involving patients and families in care and listening to their needs. It is also important to remain aware of the fact that for many people hospital care is the only option and for some the preferred choice for those who have limited resources to care for dying relatives at home. Hospitals and hospices offer patients and families security as well as the opportunity of professional help and support. In both contexts where care has been provided at home prior to admission, changes take place in the role of the carer and the care provider. Sensitive and compassionate nursing assessment involves seeking family involvement at an early stage during admission to the institution. If the patient is likely to die at home, it is imperative that the family have contact numbers and receive a rapid response if either the patient or relatives become distressed.

The need for continuity

Another important part of the care of dying patients admitted for short term care, such as respite care or symptom control, is the importance of liaising with the referring unit to ensure adequate information is passed on. During the many years at Cedar House and Newlands (Chapters 6 and 7) a number of residents were hospitalised for a variety of reasons such as falls or minor surgical operations such as hernia or varicose vein operations. The manager of Cedar House pointed out how, after a period of time in hospital, residents returned feeling disorientated and depressed. Some had developed infections and were discharged with pressure sores due in part to the change of context. Nurses in hospital should be aware of the need to maintain liaison with other colleagues in residential and nursing homes in order to be informed of the patients' individual needs and attempt where possible to ensure a high degree of continuity between each of the care contexts.

Unpopular dying patients

A particular concern regarding institutional care is the changes patients undergo as their stay increases, often referred to as institutionalisation. This is a process which can also affect the staff of many establishments. Institutions like hospitals require the patient to adopt a passive role in order to conform to the various regimes and adapt to the hospital routine. Nurses caring for dying patients need to be aware of the extent to which terminally ill patients can be changed or pacified by the process of dying (or in some cases exhibit aggressive behaviour and become uncharacteristically garrulous). In most cases patients facing impending death are generally recognised as being very vulnerable. It is also important to become aware of the perception that other staff have of such patients and in particular, become aware of the negative influence of the patient becoming unpopular. In my hospital study this became a problem for a dying patient (referred to as David in Chapter 3). David was a difficult patient to look after and was often ill-mannered, bad tempered and miserable. This did not endear him to the staff who regarded him as a miserable patient and adopted a variety of avoidance tactics to limit the extent to which he could be unpleasant towards them. Others have found that unpopular patients can have negative experiences of hospital care (Johnson 1993). The challenge for professional nursing care in relation to caring for dying patients is to ensure that the patient is protected from adverse prejudice and to utilise research evidence on unpopular patients (such as Johnson's), to draw attention to situations where the patient and the family can receive poor standards of care when they are in such a vulnerable position. Care in the hospital context often requires patients to abdicate responsibility for care to professionals and for patients to adopt the sick role. This can be both a desirable one for the patient as well as a difficult process, especially when the family are not satisfied that the care being given is of a sufficient standard or where the care is below what the patient is used to receiving at home. Conversely, the patient who is admitted to hospital or hospice because the family were unable to cope at home may experience and share a sense of relief and gratitude that their burden has been lifted.

The importance of context

The context in which many patients are cared for influences their quality of life and in many cases the treatment outcome. The role of the nurse in caring for dying patients at the end of life largely rests on their ability to exercise compassion and integrity bringing both skills to the fore, especially when ethical issues such as withdrawing treatment, CPR, DNR and withholding hydration are being discussed. Being a patient on Intensive Care is a different experience to being on an older person's ward, a labour ward or a children's unit where the 'care culture' is constantly being negotiated and reformulated by nurses and doctors who make up, develop and maintain the culture. It is important for nurses in any context of care to ensure that the dying individual is allowed to develop their own sense of uniqueness. Therefore, it requires the nurse to ensure that patients are allowed to express views and that empowerment of the patient shifts from being a trendy buzz-word to a practical reality. Feeling part of the context in which care is given is essential for personal growth, it is also, many would argue, their individual right (Kendrick 1991). Ensuring patient autonomy goes a long way towards providing the key components of a good death namely personal dignity, respect for the person and quality of life. It is also an essential part of palliative care. When cure is no longer the aim of treatment the role of the nurse in caring for the dying person needs to focus on striving to ensure that the individuality of the person is maintained and that they play an active role in the care culture. When the context determines that the dying person's role becomes secondary, it is time to change the culture and the people that make up that culture, so that the primary goal of care is the maximisation of the dying person's quality of life. In some contexts such as hospitals, where the primary aim of care is not to carry out palliative care, this goal becomes problematic. The challenge for professional caregivers in such settings is to ensure that they enable the dying patient and the family to have a voice. This voice should be listened to and the response based on meeting the needs of the person and not the context in which the care is being provided.

Summary

This chapter has reviewed and expanded upon much of what has been described and discussed in previous chapters. The experience of dying in any given context is complex and inter-subjective. It is influenced by: the individual; the family; the disease process; and the carer's ability to provide optimal treatment and care. The experience of dying is also closely associated with quality of life, which is subjective and often can only be measured by what the dying person is feeling and telling us at any given time. It is dynamic and also capable of being influenced by the setting and the people within it. At the end of life the quality of dying is linked to the way in which the five Cs (compassion, conscience, commitment, competence and confidence) are demonstrated through empathy for the person and their experience. Only when we can ensure the patient's voice is heard despite the constraints placed on them by the context of care, can we be sure that the goals of palliative care for dying people are being achieved.

Further reading

Ahmedzai S. (1993) 'The medicalisation of dying: a doctor's view' in Clark D. (ed) *The future for palliative care*. Open University Press, Buckingham: 140–7.

This essay forms part of a chapter on the medicalisation of dying and provides some very insightful comments from a hospice medical director about the role of medicine in palliative care in general and doctors in hospices particularly. Ahmedzai discusses the unhealthy obsessions of medicine with pain control and discusses the drug control exerted over patients with cancer symptoms.

Biswas B. (1993) 'The medicalisation of dying: a nurse's view' in Clark D. (ed) *The future for palliative care*. Open University Press, Buckingham: 132–9.

Biswas discusses the development of the hospice movement and clearly defines what is meant by medicalisation in the hospice context. An interesting part of the chapter is the discussion on palliative care and terminal care, which the author points out, are not synonymous.

Field D. (1994) 'Palliative medicine and the medicalisation of death'. *European Journal of Cancer Care* 3, 58–62.

This is a very interesting article, which adopts a critical view of the role of palliative medicine as a specialty and its role in the care of dying patients. Field expresses a number of concerns: a lack of clarity about the remit of medicine; the shift away from terminal care; and the inappropriate use of medical technology and the consequences and implications for hospice care of increasing medicalisation. The article is an interesting and lively part of the debate concerning medicine's role in palliative care and the role of hospices as elitist centres of care.

Useful contacts

Alzheimer's Society
Gordon House
10 Greencoat Place
London SW1P 1PH
Tel: 020 7306 0606
Membership hotline: 0845 306 0868
www.alzheimers.org.uk

Association for Death Education and Counseling (ADEC)
342 North Main St
West Hartford CT 061172507
01 (860) 586–7503
www.adec.org

Breast Cancer Care
Kiln House
210 New Kings Rd
London SW6 4NZ
Tel: 020 7384 2984
Helpline: 0808 800 60000
(textphone 0808 8006001)

British Association of Cancer United Patients (Cancer BACUP)
3 Bath Place Rivington St
London EC2A 3JR
020 7696 9003
Local centres throughout Britain
Helpline: 0808 800 1234
Professional contact: Elizabeth Lodge Partnerships Manager
Tel: 020 7920 7258
www.cancerbacup.org.uk

British Association for Counselling and Psychotherapy
BACP House, 35–37 Albert St

Rugby, CV21 2SG.
Tel: 0870 443 5252
E mail: bacp@bacp.co.uk
www.bacp.co.uk

British Humanist Society
(Funerals without God)
1 Gower Street
London WC1E 6HD
Tel: 020 7079 3580
www.humanism.org.uk

Cot Death Society
4 West Mills Yard
Kennet Rd, Newbury
Berks, RG14 5LP
Tel: 01635 38137
Monitor helpline: 0845 6010234
Email@ fundraising@
cotdeathsociety.org.uk
www.cotdeathsociety.org.uk

Counsel and Care
(Help and advice for older people)
Advice Work Dept
Twyman House
16 Bonny Street
London NW1 9PG
Tel: 0845 300 7585
Email: advice@counselandcare.org.uk
www.counselandcare.org.uk

Cruse Bereavement Care
Cruse House 126 Sheen Rd
Richmond
Surrey TW9 1UR
Tel: 020 8939 9552

Helpline: 08701671677
Email:
helpline@crusebereavement
care.org.uk

**Foundation for the Study of
Infant Deaths (FSID)**
Artillery House
London
SW1P IRT
Tel: 0870 787 0885
Helpline: 0870 787 0554
E mail: fsid@sids.org.uk
www.sids.org.uk

Help the Hospices
Hospice House
34–44 Brittania St
London WC1X 9JG
Tel +44 (0)20 7278 1021
www.helpthehospices.org.uk

Hospice Information Service
St Christopher's hospice
51–59 Lawrie Park Rd
Sydenham London
SE26 6DZ
Tel: 0870 903 3903
www.hospiceinformation.info/

**Lesbian and Gay Bereavement
Project**
Vaughan Williams Centre
Colingdale hospital
Colingdale Avenue
London
NW9 5HG
Tel: 0208 200 0511
Email: LGBP@aol.com
Helpline: 0208 8455 8894
Website: www.directions-
plus.org.uk

Macmillan Cancer Relief
(Macmillan Nurses)
89 Albert Embankment
London SE1 7UR
Tel: 020 7840 7840
Macmillan Cancerline: 0808
8082020
www.macmillan.org.uk

Marie Curie Cancer Care
89 Albert Embankment
London
SE1 7TP
Tel: 020 7599 7777
Offices in Wales, Scotland
and Northern Ireland
www.mariecurie.org.uk

**Motor Neurone Disease
Society**
PO box 246
Northampton, NN1 2
Tel: 01604 250505
Helpline: 08457 626262
E mail:
enquiries@mndassociation.org

**National Multiple Sclerosis
(MS) Society**
372 Edgeware Rd
London NW2 6ND
Tel: 020 8438 0700
Centres throughout UK
Free MS helpline
www.mssociety.org.uk

**National Association of
Bereavement Services**
2nd Floor
4 Pinchin St
London E1 1SA
Tel: 020 7709 9090

National Association of Widows
48 Queens Rd
Coventry
CV1 3EH
Tel: 024 7663 4848
www.widows.uk.net

Shadow of Suicide
(Help and advice)
109 Abbeyville Rd
London SW4 8LJ
Tel: 0171 622 7932

Still Birth and Neonatal Death Society
(SANDS)
28 Portland Place,
London W1B 1LY
Tel: 020 7436 7940
Helpline: 020 7436 5881
support@uk-sands.org
www.uk-sands.org/top.html

Terence Higgins Trust
(HIV & AIDS charity)
52–54 Gray's Inn
London WC1 8JU
Tel: 020 78310330
Regional centres in England
Direct Helpline 0845 1221 200
Email: info@tht.org.uk
www.tht.org.uk

The Compassionate Friends UK (TCP)
(Support for bereaved parents and their families)
53 North Street

Bristol BS3 1EN
Tel: 08451 20 37 85
Information and support:
info@tcf.org.uk
Helpline: 08451 23 23 04
www.tcf.org.uk

The Grief Centre
362 Manchester Rd
Droylsden
Manchester
M43 6QX
Tel: 0161 371 8860
E mail: grief@mabf.org.uk
www.mabf.org.uk

The Natural Death Centre
6 Blackstock Mews
Blackstock rd
London N4 2BT
Tel: +44 (0) 871 288 2098
www.naturaldeath.org.uk

The Patients Association
(NHS patients, advice and support)
PO Box 935
Harrow, Middlesex
HA1 3YJ
Tel: 020 8423 9100
Helpline: 08456 084455

The Samaritans
08457 90 90 90 (UK)
1850 60 90 90 (ROI)
Local branches throughout the country
Email: jo@samaritans.org

References

Abu-Saad H. (2001) *Evidence based palliative care: across the life span.* Blackwell Science, London.

Ackroyd S. (1993) 'Towards an understanding of nurses' attachments to their work: morale amongst nurses in an acute hospital'. *Journal of Advances in Health and Nursing Care* 2 (3), 23–45.

Addington-Hall J. M. & Higginson I. (eds) (2001) *Palliative Care for Non-Cancer Patients.* Oxford University Press, Oxford.

Addington-Hall J.M., Fhoury W. & McCarthy M. (1998) 'Palliative care in non-malignant disease'. *Palliative Medicine* 12 (6), 417–28.

Ahmedzai S. (1993) 'The medicalisation of dying: a doctor's view' in Clark D. (1993) *The future for palliative care.* Open University Press, Buckingham: 140–7.

Appleton M. (1995) *At home with terminal illness – a family guide to hospice at home.* Prentice Hall, New England.

Archer J. (2001) 'Grief from an evolutionary perspective' in Stroebe M.S., Hansson R.O., Stroebe W. & Schut H. (eds) *Handbook of bereavement research.* American Psychological Society, Washington DC: 263–84.

Aries P. (1974) *Western attitudes towards death.* Harvard University Press, Baltimore.

Armstrong D. (1983) 'The fabrication of nurse-patient relationships'. *Social science and Medicine* 17 (8), 651–7.

Aspinall F., Addington-Hall J., Hughes Rhidian & Higginson I.J. (2003) 'Using satisfaction to measure the quality of palliative care: a review of the literature'. *Journal of Advanced Nursing* 42 (4), 324–39.

Axelsson B. & Sjoden P.O. (1998) 'Quality of life of cancer patients and their spouses in palliative care homes'. *Palliative Medicine* 12, 29–39.

Baker D.E. (1978) *Attitudes of nurses towards elderly care.* Unpublished PhD thesis, University of Manchester, UK.

Battin M.P. (1989) 'Euthanasia is ethical' in Bernards N. (ed) *Euthanasia: Opposing viewpoints.* Greenhaven Press, San Diego.

Bauman Z. (1992) *Mortality, Immortality and other life strategies.* Polity Press, London.

Berger P. & Luckmann T. (1991) *The Social Construction of Reality.* Penguin, London (originally published in 1967).

Bhaskar K. (1979) *The possibility of naturalism: a philosophical critique of the human sciences.* Harvester Wheatsheaf, Hertfordshire.

Biswas B. (1993) 'The medicalisation of dying: a nurse's view' in: Clark D. (ed) *The future for palliative care.* OU Press, Buckingham: 132–9.

Black J. (1991) 'Death and bereavement: the customs of Hindus, Sikhs and Muslims'. *Bereavement Care* (10)1, 6–8.

Booth K., Luker K.A., Costello J. & Dows K. (2003) 'Specialist nurses in cancer and palliative care: their practice development support needs'. *International Journal of Palliative Nursing* 9(2), 73–9.

Bos M. (2003) 'Not the hospital. Not the hospital!' in Buijssen H. & Bruntink R. (eds) *A good ending, good for all?* Steil/Tred Publishers, Tilburg and Nijmegen Netherlands: 33–8.

Bowman G.S. & Thompson D.R. (1995) 'Strategies for organising care' in Schober J.E. & Hinchliff S.M. (eds) *Towards advanced nursing practice.* Arnold, London: 222–51.

Brechin A. (1998) 'Introduction' in *Care matters.* Brechin A., Walmsley J. & Katz J. (eds) Sage, London.

Brykczynska G. (1992) 'Caring – a dying art?' in Jolley M. & Brykczynska G. (eds) *Nursing care: The challenge to change.* Edward Arnold, London: 1–45.

Buckingham R.W., Lack S.A., Mount B.M., Maclean L.D. & Collins J.T. (1976) 'Living with the dead: use of the technique of participant observation'. *Canadian Medical Association Journal* 115, 1211–15.

Carson M., Williams T., Everett A. & Barker S. (1997) 'The nurse's role in the multidisciplinary team'. *European Journal of Palliative care* 4(3), 96–8.

Cartwright A. (1991) 'Balance of care for the dying between hospitals and the community: perceptions of general practitioners, hospital consultants, community nurses and relatives'. *British Journal of General Practice* 41, 348, 271–4.

Cassell E.J. (1991) *The nature of suffering and the goals of medicine.* Oxford University Press, New York.

Chassin M.R. (1996) 'Quality of health care – improving the quality of care'. *New England Journal of Medicine* 335, 14, 1060–63.

Clark D. (1993) 'Wither the hospices' in Clark D. (ed) *The future for palliative care.* OU Press Buckingham: 167–77.

Clark D. (2000) 'Death in Staithes' in Dickenson D., Johnson M. & Katz J.S. (eds) *Death, Dying and Bereavement,* (2nd editon). Open University Press, Buckingham: 1–3.

Clark D. (2002) 'Between hope and acceptance: the medicalisation of dying'. *British Medical Journal* 324, 905–7.

Clark D. (2002a) *The space for death.* Keynote paper to the 19th International Conference on Death, Dying and Bereavement York, UK.

Clark D. & Seymour J. (1999) *Reflections on palliative care.* Open University Press, Buckingham.

Cobb M. (2001) *The dying soul: spiritual care at the end of life.* OU Books, Buckingham.

Cohen G.L (1964) *What's wrong with hospitals?* Penquin, London.

Cooke H. (2000) *When someone dies: a practical guide to holistic care at the end of life*. Butterworth, Heinemann, Oxford, UK.

Copp G. (1999) *Facing impending death*. NT Books, London.

Corner J. & Dunlop R. (1997) 'New approaches to care' in Clark D., Hockley J. & Ahmedzai S. (eds) *New Themes in Palliative Care*. OU Press, Buckingham: 288–302.

Costello J. (1990) 'Dying at home'. *Nursing Times* 86(8), 49–51.

Costello J. (1994) 'The role of the nurse in the multidisciplinary team'. *Reviews in Clinical Gerontology* 4, 169–76.

Costello J. (1996) 'Acknowledging loss: Reflections on bereavement'. *Elderly Care* 8(4), 35–6.

Costello J. (1999) 'Anticipatory grief: coping with the impending death of a partner'. *International Journal of Palliative Nursing* 5 (5), 223–31.

Costello J. (2000) *Dying in a public place: ethnography of terminal care for older people in hospital*. Unpublished PhD thesis. Manchester Metropolitan University, Manchester, UK.

Costello J. (2000a) 'Truth telling and the dying patient: a silent conspiracy'. *International Journal of Palliative Nursing* 6 (8), 152–8.

Costello J. (2002) 'Do Not Resuscitate orders and older patients: findings from an ethnographic study of hospital wards for older people'. *Journal of Advanced Nursing* 39 (5), 491–9.

Costello J. & Horne M. (2003) 'Nurses' and Health Support Workers' views on CPR in a hospice setting'. *International Journal of Palliative Nursing* 9(5), 157–65.

Counsel and Care (1995) *Last rights: a study of how death and dying are handled in residential and nursing homes*. Counsel and Care, London.

Currie L. (1998) *Directory of UK Trusts using care pathways*. RCN Institute, Oxford.

Davidson B., Degner L. & Morgan T. (1995) 'Information and decision making preferences of men with prostate cancer'. *Oncology Nursing Forum* 22 (9), 1401–8.

Department of Health (DoH) (1987) HC(87)4(2). DoH, London.

Department of Health (DoH) (1990) *The NHS and Community Care Act*. DoH, London.

Department of Health (DoH) (1995) Calman K. & Hine D.A. *A policy framework for commissioning cancer services: Report by the expert advisory group on cancer to the Chief Medical Officer*, London.

Department of Health (DoH) (1997) *The New NHS: Modern, Dependable*. HMSO cm 3807. The Stationery Office, London.

Department of Health (DoH) (2000) *The NHS Cancer Plan. A plan for investment. A plan for reform*, London.

Department of Health (DoH) (2000a) *The Care Standards Act*. DoH, London.

Department of Health (DoH) (2001) *National Service Framework for Older People*. DoH, London.

Department of Health (DoH) (2002) *Care homes for older people: national minimum standards and care home regulations* (2nd edition). DoH, London.

Department of Social Security (DSS) (2000) *A guide to benefits*. DSS Communications. Belmont Press, Leeds.

Department of Social Security (2000a) *What to do after a death in England and Wales*. DSS Communications. Belmont Press, Leeds.

Diver F., Molassiotis A. & Weeks L. (2003) 'The palliative care needs of ethnic minority patients attending a day care centre: a qualitative study'. *International Journal of Palliative Nursing* 9 (9), 389–96.

Douglas C (1992) 'For all the saints'. *British Medical Journal* 304, 579.

Douglas M. (ed) (1977) *Rules and Meanings*. Penguin, London.

Doyle D. (1994) 'The future of palliative care' in Corless I.B., Germino B.B. & Pittman M. (eds) *Dying, death and bereavement: theoretical perspectives and other ways of knowing*. Jones & Bartlett, Boston and London.

Dunphy K.P. & Amesbury B.D.W. (1990) 'A comparison of hospice and home care patients: patients of referral, patient characteristics and predictors of place of death'. *Palliative Medicine* 4, 105–11.

Ellershaw J. (2001) Paper given to the Trans Pennine palliative care research network conference Cheadle Cheshire 'The challenge of transferring hospice philosophy to hospitals'. 13 June, St Ann's Hospice.

Ellershaw J. & Murphy D. (2003) 'The national pathway network of palliative care pathways'. *Journal of Integrated Care Pathways* 7, (1)3–11.

Ellershaw J. & Wilkinson S. (2003) *Care of the dying: a pathway to excellence*. Oxford University Press, Oxford.

Ellershaw J., Foster A., Murphy D., Shea T. & Overill S. (1997) 'Developing an Integrated Care Pathway for the dying patient'. *European Journal of Palliative Care* 4 (6), 203–7.

Etzioni, A. (1964) *Modern organisations*. Prentice Hall, Englewood Cliffs NJ.

Eve A. & Smith A.E. (1996) 'Survey of hospice and palliative care inpatient units in the UK and Ireland'. *Palliative Medicine* 10 (1), 13–21.

Evers H.K. (1981) 'Multidisciplinary teams in geriatric wards: myth or reality?'. *Journal of Advanced Nursing* 6, 205–14.

Fallowfield L. (1995) 'Psychosocial interventions in cancer should be part of every patient's management plan'. *British Medical Journal* 311(7016), 1316–17.

Faull C. & Woof R. (2002) *Palliative care*. Oxford University Press, Oxford.

Feifel H. (1959) *The meaning of death*. McGraw-Hill, New York.

Field D. (1984) 'We didn't want him to die on his own': nurses' accounts of nursing dying patients'. *Journal of Advanced Nursing* 9, 59–70.

Field D. (1987) *Opening up awareness: nurses' accounts of nursing the dying.* Unpublished Ph.D. thesis, University of Leicester, UK.

Field D. (1989) *Nursing the dying.* Routledge, London.

Field D. (1994) 'Palliative medicine and the medicalisation of death'. *European Journal of Cancer Care* 3, 58–62.

Field D. (1998) 'Special not different: General Practitioners' accounts of their care of dying people'. *Social Science and Medicine* 46 (9), 111–1120.

Field D. & Copp G. (1999) 'Communication and awareness about dying in the 1990s'. *Palliative Medicine* 13(6), 459–68.

Field D. & Froggatt K. (2003) 'Issues for palliative care in nursing and residential care homes' in Peace S. & Katz J.S. *End of life in care homes.* Oxford University Press, Oxford, UK: 175–94.

Field, D. & James, N. (1993) 'Where and how people die' in Clark D. (ed) *The future for palliative care.* Open University Press, Buckingham: 6–29.

Field M.J. & Cassell C.K. (eds) (1997) *Approaching death: improving care at the end of life.* National Academy Press, Washington DC: 24.

Flax J. (1990) *Thinking fragments.* University of California Press, Berkeley.

Ford P. & Heath H. (1996) *Older people and nursing: issues of living in a care home.* Butterworth Heinemann, London.

Foucault M. (1970) *The order of things.* Tavistock, London.

Fox N. (1993) *Post-modernism, sociology and health.* OU Press, Buckingham.

Froggatt K. (2000) 'Evaluating a palliative care pilot project in nursing homes'. *International Journal of Palliative Nursing* 6, 140–6.

Froggatt K. (2001) 'Palliative care and nursing homes: where next?' *Palliative Medicine* 15, 42–8.

Froggatt K., Hoult L. & Poole K. (2001) *Community work with nursing and residential care homes: a survey study of clinical nurse specialists in palliative care.* Macmillan Cancer Relief/The Institute of Cancer Research, London.

Garrett G. (1994) *Healthy ageing.* Wolfe Publishing, London.

Giddens A. (1997) *Sociology* (3rd edition). Polity Press, London.

Glaser B.G. & Strauss A.L. (1965) *Awareness of dying.* Aldine Publishing, Chicago.

Glaser B.G. & Strauss A.L. (1968) *Time for Dying.* Aldine Publishing, Chicago.

Goffman E. (1968) *Asylums.* Pelican, London.

Gorer G. (1987) (reprint) *Death, Grief and Mourning in Contemporary Britain.* Ayer Publishers, Salem, New Hampshire.

Grbich C. (2003) *New approaches in social research*. Sage, London.

Griffin A.P. (1981) 'A philosophical analysis of caring in nursing'. *Journal of Advanced Nursing* 8 (4), 289–95.

Health Advisory Service (HAS) (2000) *Not because they are old*. HAS, DoH, London.

Higginson I.J., Astin P. & Dolan S. (1998) 'Where do cancer patients die? Ten year trends in the place of death of cancer patients in England'. *Palliative Medicine* 12, 353–63.

Higginson I.J., Finlay J., Goodwin D.M., Cook A.M., Hood K., Edwards A.G.K., Douglas H. & Norman C.E. (2002) 'Do hospital based palliative care teams improve care for patients at the end of life?' *Journal of Pain and Symptom Management* 23 (2), 96–106.

Hill A. (1998) 'Multi-professional teamwork in hospital palliative care teams'. *International Journal of Palliative Nursing* 4 (5), 214–21.

Hindmarch C. (2000) *On the death of a child* (2nd edition). Radcliffe Medical Press, Abingdon Oxon.

Hinton J. (1972) *Dying*. Penguin Books, London.

Hockey J. (1990) *Experiences of death: an anthropological account*. Edinburgh University Press, Edinburgh.

Hockley J.M., Dunlop R. & Davies R.J. (1988) 'Survey of distressing symptoms in dying patients and their families in hospital in response to a symptom control team'. *British Medical Journal* 296, 1715–17.

Hockley L. (1997) 'The evolution of the hospice approach' in Clark D., Hockley J. & Ahmedzai S. *New themes in palliative care*. OU Press, Buckingham: 84–100.

Honeybun, J., Johnston M. & Tookman A. (1992) 'The impact of a death on fellow Hospice patients'. *British Journal of Medical Psychology* 65, 67–72.

Hopkinson J.B. (2002) 'Facilitating the development of clinical skills in caring for dying people in hospital'. *Nurse Education Today* 21, 632–39.

Hunt M. (1991) 'The identification and provision of care for the terminally ill at home by family members'. *Sociology of Health and Illness* 13 (3), 373–95.

Hunt M. (1991a) 'Being friendly and informal: reflected in nurses', terminally ill patients' and relatives' conversations at home'. *Journal of Advanced Nursing* 16, 929–38.

Illich I. (1990) *Limits to medicine: medical nemesis the expropriation of health*. Penguin, London.

Irvine B. (1993) 'Development in palliative nursing in and out of the hospital setting'. *British Journal of Nursing* 3 (4), 218–20.

Jack B., Oldham J. & Williams A. (2002) 'Do hospital based palliative care nurse specialists de-skill general staff?'. *International Journal of Palliative Nursing* 8 (7), 336–40.

Jack B.A., Gambles M., Murphy D. & Ellershaw J.E. (2003) 'Nurses' perceptions of the Liverpool Care Pathway for the dying patient in the acute hospital setting'. *International Journal of Palliative Nursing* 9 (9), 375–81.

James N & Field D (1996) 'Who has the power? Some problems and issues affecting the nursing care of dying patients'. *European Journal of Cancer Care* 5, 73–80.

James V. (1986) *Care and work in nursing the dying: a participant study in a continuing care unit.* Unpublished Ph.D. thesis, University of Aberdeen, UK.

Johnson I.S. Rogers R., Biswas B. & Ahmedzai S. (1990) 'What do hospices do? A survey of hospices in the United Kingdom'. *British Medical Journal* 300, 24 March, 791–93.

Johnson M. (1993) *Unpopular patients reconsidered: an interpretive ethnography of the process of social judgment in a hospital ward.* Unpublished Ph.D. thesis, University of Manchester, UK.

Jolley M. & Brykczynska G. (1992) *Nursing care: the challenge to care.* Arnold, London.

Jones R.V.H. (1992) 'Primary health care: what should we do for people dying at home from cancer?'. *European Journal of Cancer Care* 1, 9–11.

Jones R.V.H., Hansford J. & Fiske J. (1993) 'Death from cancer at home: the carers' perspective'. *British Medical Journal* 306, 249–51.

Jupp P.C. & Gittings C. (eds) (1999) *Death in England: an illustrated history.* Manchester University Press, Manchester.

Kastenbaum R. (1982) 'New fantasies in the American death system'. *Death Education* 6, 155–66.

Kastenbaum R. (1995) *Death, Society and Human Experience.* Allyn & Bacon, Boston, USA.

Kastenbaum R. (1996) 'World without death'. *Mortality* 1(1), 11–22.

Katz J. & Sidell M. (1994) *Easeful Death.* Hodder & Stoughton, London.

Katz J., Komaromy C. & Sidell M. (1995) *Death and dying in residential and nursing homes for older people – examining the case for palliative care.* Report for the Department of Health. London.

Katz J.S. & Peace S. (2003) *End of life in care homes: a palliative care approach.* Oxford University Press, Oxford.

Keady J. (1997) 'Relatives' views of care in residential/nursing homes'. *British Journal of Nursing* 6, 11, 606.

Kearl M.C. (1989) *Endings: a sociology of death and dying.* Oxford University Press, Oxford.

Kellehear A. (1992) *Dying of Cancer: the final year of life.* Harwood Academic Press, Switzerland.

Kellehear A. (1999) *Health promoting palliative care.* Oxford University Press, Oxford, UK.

Kellner B. (1988) 'Post-modernism as social theory: some challenges and problems'. *Theory, Culture and Society* 5, 239–70.

Kendrick K. (1991) 'Partners in passing: ethical aspects of nursing the dying person'. *Journal of Advances in Health and Nursing Care* 1 (1), 11–27.

King Edward's Hospital Fund for London and the National Association of Health Authorities and Trusts (1991) *Care of the dying: a guide for health authorities.* NAHA, Birmingham.

Kite S. (1997) 'How can different models of organisation or bed utilisation improve the care of patients dying in hospital?' in Bosanquet N., Kilbery C., Salisbury P., Franks S., Kite S., Lorentzon M. et al (eds) *Appropriate and cost effective models of service delivery in palliative care.* London Dept of Primary Health Care and General Practice, Imperial School of Medicine at St Mary's.

Klein R. (1998) *The new politics of the NHS.* Longman, London.

Kubler-Ross, E. (1970) *On death and dying.* New York, Macmillan.

Lawler J. (1991) *Behind the screens: nursing, somology, and the problem of the body.* Churchill Livingstone, London.

Lawton J. (2000) *The dying process: patients' experiences of palliative care.* Routledge, London.

Lee E. (1995) *A good death: a guide for patients and carers facing terminal illness at home.* Rosendale Press, London.

Leese D. (2002) 'Book review: Integrated Care Pathways: a practical approach to implementation'. *Nurse Education Today* 21, 502–3.

Lemert C. (1992) 'General social theory, irony, post-modernism' in Seidman S. & Wagner D. (eds) *Post-modernism and social theory.* Blackwell, Oxford.

Levi-Strauss C. (1968) *Structural anthropology.* Penguin Press, London.

Lewis, C.S. (1961) *A Grief Observed.* Faber and Faber, London.

Littlewood J. (1992) *Aspects of grief: bereavement in adult life.* Routledge, London.

Logue B.J. (1994) 'When Hospice Fails: The limits of Palliative Care' *Omega* 29 (4), 291–301.

Luker K., Beaver K., Austin L. & Leinster S.J. (2002) 'An evaluation of information cards as a means of improving communication between hospital and primary care for women with breast cancer'. *Journal of Advanced Nursing* 31 (5), 1174–82.

Luker K., Beaver K., Leinster S. & Owens R. (1996) 'Information needs and sources of information for women with breast cancer: a follow up study'. *Journal of Advanced Nursing* 23, 487–95.

Lupton D. (1995) 'Perspectives on power, communication and the medical encounter: implications for nursing theory and practice'. *Nursing Inquiry* 2, 157–63.

Lynch M. & Abrahm J. (2002) 'Ensuring a good death'. *Cancer Practice* 10 (1), 33–9.

Mackay L. (1989) *Nursing a problem*. Open University Press, Buckingham, 37–54.

Mackay L. (1993) *Conflicts in care: medicine and nursing*. Chapman & Hall, London.

Maddocks I. (1996) 'Palliative care in the nursing home'. *Progress in Palliative care*, 4, 77–8.

Maddocks I. & Parker D. (2001) 'Palliative care in nursing homes' in Addington-Hall J. & Higginson I. (eds) *Palliative care for non-cancer patients*. Oxford University Press, Oxford: 147–57.

Mallik M. (1997) 'Advocacy in nursing: a review of the literature'. *Journal of Advanced Nursing* 25, 130–8.

May C. (1992) 'Individual care? Power and subjectivity in therapeutic relationships'. *Sociology* 26(4), 589–602.

May C. (1993) 'Subjectivity and culpability in the constitution of nurse-patient relationships'. *International Journal of Nursing Studies* 30(2), 181–92.

May, C. (1995) 'Patient autonomy and the politics of professional relationships'. *Journal of Advanced Nursing* 21, 83–7.

McIntosh J. (1977) *Communication and awareness in a cancer ward*. Croom Helm, London.

McNamara B. (2001) *Fragile lives: death dying and care*. Open University Press, Buckingham.

McNamara B., Waddell C. & Colvin M. (1994) 'The institutionalisation of the good death'. *Social Science and Medicine* 39, 11, 1501–8.

Miller A. (1985) 'Nurse-patient dependency – is it iatrogenic?'. *Journal of Advanced Nursing* 10, 63–9.

Miller E.J. & Gwynne G.V. (1972) *A life apart: a pilot study of residential institutions for the physically handicapped and the very young sick*. Tavistock Books, London.

Miller R.J. (1992) 'Hospice care as an alternative to euthanasia'. *Law, Medicine and Health Care* 20, 127–32.

Mills M., Davies H.T.O. & Macrae W.A. (1994) 'Care of dying patients in hospital'. *British Medical Journal* 309, September, 583–6.

Miskella C. & Avis M. (1998) 'Care of the dying person in the nursing home: exploring the care assistants' contribution'. *European Journal of Oncology Nursing* 2 (2), 80–6.

Moss M. & Moss S. (1996) 'The impact of family deaths on older people'. *Bereavement Care* 15 (3), 26–7.

National Association of Health Authorities and Trusts (1991) *Care of people with terminal illness*. National Association of Health Authorities and Trusts, Birmingham.

National Council for Hospice and Specialist Palliative Care Services (NCHSPCS) (1995) *Opening doors: Improving access to hospice and specialist palliative care services by members of the black and ethnic minority communities.* Occasional Paper 7. NCHSPCS, London.

National Council for Hospice and Specialist Palliative Care Services (NCHSPCS) (1996) *Palliative Care in the Hospital Setting.* Occasional Paper 10, NCHSPCS, London.

National Council for Hospice and Specialist Palliative Care Services (NCHSPCS) (1997) *Making Palliative Care Better.* Occasional Paper 12. NCHSPCS, London.

Neuberger J. (1987) *Caring for dying patients of different faiths.* Sainsbury series, Austin Cornish, London.

Newton E. (1980) *This bed my centre.* Virago, London.

ONS Office of National Statistics (2000) http://www.statistics.gov.uk

Overill S. (1998) 'A practical guide to care pathways'. *Journal of Integrated Care* 2, 93–8.

Ovretveit J. (1995) 'Team decision making'. *Journal of Inter-professional Care* 9 (1), 41–51.

Parkes C.M. (1972) *Bereavement: studies of grief in adult life.* Penguin, London.

Parkes C.M. (1978) 'Home or Hospital? Terminal Care as seen by surviving spouses'. *Journal of the Royal College of General Practitioners* 28, 19–30.

Parkes C.M. & Parkes J. (1984) ' "Hospice" versus "hospital" care re-evaluation after 10 years as seen by surviving spouses'. *Post-Graduate Medical Journal* 60, 120–24.

Parkes C.M., Relf M. & Couldrick A. (1996) *Counselling in terminal care and bereavement.* British Psychological Society, London.

Payne S., Hillier R., Langley-Evans A. & Roberts T. (1996) 'Impact of witnessing death on hospice patients'. *Social Science and Medicine* 43 (12), 1785–94.

Peace S. & Katz J.S. (2003) 'End of life in care homes' in Katz J.S. & Peace S. (eds) *End of life in care homes: a palliative care approach.* Oxford University Press, Oxford: 195–200.

Peace S., Kellaher L. & Willcocks D. (1997) *Re-evaluating Residential Care.* Open University Press, Buckingham.

Pearce E. (1963) *A general textbook of nursing* (first published 1937). Faber & Faber, London.

Penson J. (1993) *Bereavement: a guide for nurses.* Chapman & Hall, London.

Porter S. (1991) 'A participant observation study of power relations between nurses and doctors in a general hospital'. *Journal of Advanced Nursing* 16, 728–35.

Rando T.A. (1986) (ed.) *Anticipatory grief and loss.* Research Press, Lexington, Massachusetts.

Revans R.W. (1974) *Hospitals, Communication, Choice and Change.* Tavistock, London.

Richies G. & Dawson P. (2000) *An intimate loneliness: supporting bereaved parents and siblings.* Open University Press, Buckingham.

Riley K. (1998) *Definition of a pathway.* National Pathways Association Newsletter, Spring.

Rogers A., Karlsen S. & Addington-Hall J. (2000) 'All the services were excellent. It is when the human element comes in that things go wrong: dissatisfaction with hospital care at the end of life'. *Journal of Advanced Nursing* 31(4), 768–74.

Rose X. (1995) *Widow's journey.* Souvenir Press, London.

Russ S.A. (1989) 'Euthanasia should not be based on quality of life' in Bernards N. (ed) *Euthanasia: opposing viewpoints.* Green Haven Press, San Diego.

Saunders C. (1970) 'The nature and management of terminal pain' in Camps F., Saunders C., Dominian J., Parkes C., Calne R.Y., Dempster W.J. & Dunstan G.R. *Matters of life and death.* Darton, Longman & Todd, London: 15–26.

Saunders C. (1988) *St Christopher's in celebration.* Hodder & Stoughton, London.

Saunders C. (1996) 'A personal therapeutic journey'. *British Medical Journal* 313, 21–28 December, 1599–1601.

Schou K.S. & Hewitson J. (1998) *Experiencing cancer.* Open University Press, Buckingham.

Scottish Office Home and Health Department (1991) *'Everybody's death should matter to somebody': a review and recommendations by a working party of the Scottish Health Service advisory council.* HMSO, London.

Scrutton S. (1995) *Bereavement and grief: supporting older people through loss.* Edward Arnold/Age Concern, London.

Seale C. (1999) 'Awareness of method: re-reading Glaser & Strauss'. *Mortality* 4 (2), 195–202.

Seale C. & Cartwright A. (1994) *The year before death.* Avebury, Aldershot, Hants.

Seale C. & Kelly M. (1997) 'A comparison of hospice and hospital care for people who die: views of surviving spouses'. *Palliative medicine* 11, 93–100.

Seale C.F. (1989) 'What happens in hospices? A review of research evidence'. *Social Science and Medicine* 28 (6), 551–9.

Seale C.F. (1991) 'Death from cancer and death from other causes: the relevance of the Hospice approach'. *Palliative Medicine* 13, 3–17.

Seymour J. (1999) 'Revisiting medicalisation and natural death'. *Social Science and Medicine* 49, 691–704.

Seymour J.E. (2001) *Critical moments – death and dying in intensive care.* OU Press, Buckingham.

Shukla R.K. (1982) 'Primary or team nursing? Two conditions determine the choice'. *Journal of Nursing Administration* 12(11), 12–15.

Sidell M., Katz. J.T. & Komaromy C. (1997) *Death and dying in residential and nursing homes for older people.* Report to the Department of Health, London.

Smith L. (1994) 'Choice and risk in the care of elderly people' in Hunt G. (ed) *Ethical issues in nursing.* Routledge, London.

Smith P. (1992) *The emotional labour of nursing.* Macmillan, London.

Soothill K., McKay L. & Webb C. (1995) *Intra-professional relations in health care.* Edward Arnold, London.

Standing Medical Advisory Committee (1980) *Terminal care: report of a working group.* HMSO, London.

Stewart A. & Dent A. (1994) *At a loss: bereavement care when a baby dies.* Bailliere Tindall, London.

Sudnow D. (1970) 'Dying in a public place' in Brim O.G., Freeman J.L., Levine S. & Scotch N.A. (eds) *The dying patient.* Russell Sage Foundation, New York: 191–208.

Sweeting H. & Gilhooley M. (1991) 'Doctor am I dead? A review of social death in modern societies'. *Omega* 24(4), 251–69.

Sykes N.P. (1992) 'Quality of care for the terminally ill: the carer's perspective'. *Palliative Medicine* 6, 227–36.

Ten Have H. (2003) *Exploring the ethical dimensions of palliative care.* Paper to the 8th Congress of the European Association for Palliative Care, The Hague.

Thomas K. (2003) *Caring for the dying at home: companions on the journey.* Radcliffe Medical Press, Abingdon.

Timmermans S. (1994) 'Dying of awareness: the theory of awareness contexts revisited'. *Sociology of Health and Illness* 16(3), 332–39.

Todd C.J., Grande G.E., Barclay S.I.G. & Farquhar M.C. (2002) 'General practitioners' and district nurses' views of hospital at home for palliative care'. *Palliative Medicine* 16, 251–4.

Turner V.W. (1967) *The Forest of Symbols: Aspects of Ndembu Ritual.* Cornell University Press, Ithaco & London, 48–111.

Vachon, M.L.S. (1987) 'Dying patients are not the real problem' in Vachon M.L.S. (ed) *Occupational Stress in the Care of the Critically ill, the Dying and the Bereaved.* Hemisphere, Washington DC: 51–74.

Van Gennep A. (1972) *The rites of passage.* University of Chicago Press, Chicago.

Walter T. (1990) *Funerals and how to improve them*. Hodder & Stoughton, London.

Walter, T. (1994) *Revival of death*. Routledge, London.

Walter T. (1999) *On bereavement – the culture of grief*. OU Press, Buckingham.

Waterlow J. (1988) 'The Waterlow card for the prevention and management of pressure sores'. *Care – Science and Practice* 6(1), 8–12.

Waters K.R. (1987) 'Team nursing'. *Nursing Practice* 1, 7–15.

Watson J. (1999) *Post-modern nursing and beyond*. Churchill Livingstone, London.

Wilkes E. (1993) 'Introduction' in Clark D. (ed) *The future for palliative care*. OU Press, Buckingham.

Wilkinson S. & Mula C. (2003) 'Communication in care of the dying' in Ellershaw J. & Wilkinson S. (eds) *Care of the dying: a pathway to excellence*. Oxford, Oxford University Press: 74–89.

Willard C. (1996) 'The nurse's role as patient advocate: obligation or imposition'. *Journal of Advanced Nursing* 24, 60–6.

Wilson D. (2000) 'End of life preferences of Canadian senior citizens with care-giving experience'. *Journal of Advanced Nursing* 31(6), 1416–21.

Wolf Z. (1988) *Nurses work: the sacred and the profane*. University of Pennsylvania, Philadelphia.

World Health Organisation (WHO) (1990) Technical report series 804. Geneva.

World Health Organisation (WHO) (2002) *Definition of palliative care* http://www5.who.int/cancer

Wright B. (1996) *Sudden death: a research base for practice*. Churchill Livingstone, London.

Wright S.G. (1986) *Building and using a model of nursing*. Edward Arnold, London.

Young M. & Cullen L. (1996) *A good death: conversations with East Londoners*. Routledge, London.

Zander K. (1998) 'Historical development of outcomes based care delivery'. *Critical Care Nursing Clinics of North America* 10, 1–11.

Index